34134 00041432 3

Leabharlann nan Eilean Siar

D0540023

WESTER

Readers are requested to take great care of the item while in their possession, and to point out any defects that they may notice in them to the Librarian.
This item should be returned on or before the latest date stamped below, but an extension of the period of loan may be granted when desired.

WITHDRAWN

DATE OF RETURN	DATE OF RETURN	DATE OF RETURN
1 0 JAN 2011	2 0 FEB 2014	
	1 2 JUL 2019	
	- 3 OCT 2019	

Praise for *A Will to* WIN

'This true story of determination and courage cannot fail to move readers'
OK Magazine

'Peterson's book chronicles not only her physical decline, but also the overwhelming psychological tsunami faced by someone with degenerative disease'
The Times

'Alice Peterson's startling account of her attempts to come to terms with a degenerative disease is both inspiring and accomplished . . . This frank account will dispel a lot of the stereotypes associated with RA and gives testament to the strength and love of a family that was unwilling to b~ defeated. At times funny and forthright this a~~ ~~shing account by a local woman will be a so~~~ of inspiration to all those who read it'
Winchester & Bishops Waltham Observer

'An engrossing book . . . deeply affecting . . . What makes Alice's book so different – and readable – is the way she intimately and honestly describes the daily effect of such a horrible disease on a normal, previously healthy young girl. The experiences in hospital, the host of different drugs and the way they changed her body, her desperate attempts to continue a normal life and not to get left behind by her healthy contemporaries, and how the disease's unpredictability made relationships with boy-friends and college flatmates so difficult; are all unflinch-ingly chronicled'
Arthritis Today

'*A Will to Win* is the moving story of [one woman's] battle to beat a crippling disease'
Sunday Post

'The book is funny, entertaining and fast-paced, with a mercilessly-close observation of everyone from the coaches at the tennis club to the officials on the court. It is so immediate that you feel you are in the car with the teenage whirlwind and her mum, Pam, as they follow the British tournament circuit'
Hampshire Chronicle

'Alice's story is not one of despair, but of hope . . . It graphically, often with dark humour, describes how she changed from being a teenage tennis star to a young woman coming to terms with an agonising disability'
Westpress.co.uk

'Brilliant and moving'
Kentish Gazette

'Alice vividly chronicles the suffering of a young girl to whom illness has paid a horrifyingly sudden call . . . but her determination not to be overwhelmed by RA comes through strongly'
Bristol Evening Post

'This is a moving account of Alice's battle against the pain and agony of this disease, and how she came to terms with the loss of her brilliant career'
Lancashire Evening Post

'Uplifting, humorous and heart-warming'
Northern Echo

ALICE PETERSON

A Will to
WIN

*A remarkable story of courage
and determination*

WESTERN ISLES
LIBRARIES
30202085
796·342

WITHDRAWN

PAN BOOKS

First published 2001 by Macmillan

This edition published 2002 by Pan Books
an imprint of Pan Macmillan Ltd
Pan Macmillan, 20 New Wharf Road, London N1 9RR
Basingstoke and Oxford
Associated companies throughout the world
www.panmacmillan.com

ISBN 0 330 48015 4

Copyright © Alice Peterson 2001

The right of Alice Peterson to be identified as the
author of this work has been asserted by her in accordance
with the Copyright, Designs and Patents Act 1988.

All rights reserved. No part of this publication may be
reproduced, stored in or introduced into a retrieval system, or
transmitted, in any form, or by any means (electronic, mechanical,
photocopying, recording or otherwise) without the prior written
permission of the publisher. Any person who does any unauthorized
act in relation to this publication may be liable to criminal
prosecution and civil claims for damages.

1 3 5 7 9 8 6 4 2

A CIP catalogue record for this book is available from
the British Library.

Typeset by SetSystems Ltd, Saffron Walden, Essex
Printed and bound in Great Britain by
Mackays of Chatham plc, Chatham, Kent

This book is sold subject to the condition that it shall not,
by way of trade or otherwise, be lent, re-sold, hired out,
or otherwise circulated without the publisher's prior consent
in any form of binding or cover other than that in which
it is published and without a similar condition including this
condition being imposed on the subsequent purchaser.

Contents

Acknowledgements

I want to thank my cousin Bella Pollen, who has helped me enormously with my writing. She told me that I must always dig deeper, tell people what it is *really* like for someone young to have an ageing disease – 'scratching the surface of emotions isn't good enough.' She taught me not to be afraid of writing the truth, giving my work a new lease of life. Her professionalism and faith in my project have been invaluable. Bella, without you, your moral support and your red-penning I would have been lost.

I will always be profoundly grateful to Charles Drazin, who gave me the conviction to carry on writing. And to Oliver and Cynthia Colman. Thank you for your encouragement and wise guidance.

To my agent, Clare Alexander. Words are hopelessly inadequate. You have made my dream come true.

To the team at Macmillan. To Mari Evans. I can't thank you enough for believing so passionately in my book and having the faith to make it happen. You are a wonderful editor.

To Nicky Hursell. Thank you for all your encouragement and the hard work that you have put into the paperback.

And Lucy Henson, you have done a great job with the publicity. Thank you.

My sister Helen, you are the best e-mail critic and my best friend.

To Bernice Crockford who has been there for me like a second mum, through thick and thin.

Love and thanks to Judith Forshaw, Jill Hickson, Mary Firebrace and Georgiana Barrowcliff who have all helped me in so many different ways.

To Dr Buchanan, Dr Henderson, Dr Rose, Professor Dieppe and the surgeons, Mr Samuel and Mr Morrison. Tessa Campbell, my physiotherapist and occupational therapists Kate Dulson and Christina Macleod, and to the many nurses and carers who have all fought hard to help me lead a more normal life.

To all at the Pinder Centre, Avington, for hydrotherapy. I have been so lucky to have you.

My cousin Emma Foale, who has given me devoted support and a wonderful holiday in her paradise home in Spain every summer for the last eight years.

To my grandmother who is a true inspiration. You are an example to us all.

Finally, Robert Cross, without him and his undying faith my first line would never have been written. You are such a special advisor and friend. And Mary, Robert's wife – thank you for supporting our project from the very beginning.

My story is a fight involving a whole range of people. It isn't only me – that pain deeply affects others is one of the most important lessons I have learnt. I want to thank all my friends and family from the bottom of my heart, to make sure they understand how vital their support and love has been.

For my mother and father

Foreword

Alice's book reminds me of my junior tennis days – the tournaments, the training, the nervous parents standing behind the court. I remember Alice being one of the best dozen or so girl players in the country in the late 1980s.

I could not believe she was struck down with rheumatoid arthritis at the age of eighteen. I do know from experience how frustrating it is when injury stops you playing your sport for a time. But at least you know the injury is only temporary. For Alice it was much worse. Her tennis came to an end; she missed the opportunity of going to America. Her life changed in every way.

I found her book moving. It opened my eyes to the pain and suffering that goes on in this world. I also found it inspiring. Who could imagine someone subjected to this continuous pain putting themselves through a university course and getting a First. It is hard to imagine being in her shoes – but if I was, I hope I would be brave enough to build my life again and not let such a cruel blow defeat me. I am sure anyone who reads her book will find themselves admiring her courage, enjoying her humour and spirit and wishing her all possible success.

Tim Henman
August 2000

Introduction

Early summer 1997, Jasmine, my miniature wire-haired dachshund, had two adorable puppies, and it was going to be heartbreaking to sell them. I begged Mum to keep them both.

'I'm sure we'll find lovely homes for them,' Mum said hopefully. 'A great friend of ours, Robert Cross, is coming over with his wife Mary and they seem quite interested in the girl. We'll bring the puppies out on to the lawn and have tea outside. It's too sunny to be indoors,' she said, handing me Boysy, the beautiful gold puppy.

'Robert, this is Alice.' Oh God, I have to make polite conversation, I thought, shaking his hand.

'Hello dear, your mother told me about the surgery on your feet. How are you feeling?' he asked, looking at my white plastered boots. I had just had an operation to remove the metatarsal joints in both feet.

I told him about the rheumatoid arthritis and my recent operation. I also started talking about my tennis and for some reason I couldn't stop talking.

'Have you ever thought about putting this down on paper?' he asked.

Mary cut in. 'Robert's a great one for writing nervous notes. Whenever something's worrying him, I find little scraps of paper around the house,' she laughed. 'He finds writing very soothing, it helps him think things through.'

'I think you should try it. I know a little about publishing,' Robert said modestly. 'I've been in the business for a while.'

Suddenly I became excited. 'Should I go on a creative writing course?' I asked.

'You could, but I think it's much better to write uninhibited by rules. Write spontaneously, from the heart. Why don't you write something and send it to me,' Robert suggested, sensing my interest. 'I'll cast a critical eye over it.' The puppy was immediately forgotten.

I fetched my old Canon Starwriter from the attic and wiped off the dust that had settled in the cracks between the keys. The polite messages flashing on the screen and the irritating bleeping noises reminded me of Bristol University and writing endless essays. It spurred me to write about my time there and I began to tap the keys with ferocity. Something came alive within me. I showed my work to Robert and he encouraged me to continue. We began to meet regularly and it was the beginning of a very special friendship.

Writing about my illness was at first hugely therapeutic. Putting down in words my anger, fear, pain and grief gave me a great sense of freedom and relief. I wrote everything down in a jumble of thoughts and it was not until I began to piece events together that I really came to understand my feelings.

The more I wrote, the more I was able to look at events objectively, see why friendships broke up, see how my mind worked and what pulled me through. It was as if I was standing outside the picture, looking in.

When I was diagnosed with rheumatoid arthritis, it seemed like the worst imaginable thing. I wished that I had never played tennis because then I would not have felt such a dreadful, harrowing sense of loss. I wanted to erase it from my memory, pretend my tennis days had never happened. However, remembering the competitions made me think not only of the excitement and the fun I had on court, but also of my dogged determination. I always had to win, second best was not good enough. It made me realize that my tennis experiences were invaluable because I have been able to channel the determination, energy and grit I had on the tennis court into battling against RA. To this day I will never give up, because my training has instilled in me the spirit to fight. Perhaps it has been my saviour.

With renewed inspiration, I dug out tennis letters, scrapbooks, programmes and photographs. Characters came alive on paper and I began to enjoy writing about my tournaments, my tennis friends, the cheats and my nervous mother darning Tom's socks while watching me play. It made me laugh and cry at the same time. Writing it all down made me want to get back in touch with Bill, my tennis coach. It brought old friendships, torn apart at university, back into my life. I was healing open wounds and reliving memories for the first time.

I began to piece the two parts of my life together to make a whole and, instead of going to sleep worrying about how I was going to feel the next day, I went to sleep planning the next chapter in my mind. I would wake up in the middle of the night with a new idea to write down. My book opened a new door. It did not take the pain away, but I had something else to think about. Writing was beginning to replace tennis, to fill a gap I thought could never be filled. I had found a project which came to mean everything to me.

Describing the deep sadness of suddenly not being able to touch my tennis racket made me feel very strongly that not enough people are aware of how life-changing arthritis can be. It is not just a few aches and twinges here and there. I no longer shrink at the word 'arthritis' in the way that I did in the early days at Bristol University, when I felt so utterly ashamed of the condition. Rather the reverse. Now, I want passionately for people to understand that arthritis can be a chronic debilitating disease affecting both young and old. The conflict between wanting to lead a teenager's life and suffering the ageing symptoms of rheumatoid arthritis came to a head at Bristol and turned my life upside down. Arthritis of any form deserves far greater recognition and attention.

Writing about the horrific pain, the medication which seemed to do nothing but harm, and the realization that I was an extreme case made me look back on the hard times and see how I had managed to come through them. I now have the chance to make something positive out of something so seemingly destructive. I hope my book will help others in similar situations.

I

The Trial: Part 1

Are you able to dress yourself, including tying shoelaces and doing buttons?

It's February 1998. I am twenty-four. I have had rheumatoid arthritis for six years.

My parents are watching me get progressively worse. I am on the waiting-list for an ankle replacement operation and I need more surgery on my right hand. Mum has to do everything for me – from pulling up my knickers to cutting my food, heaving me out of the chair and helping me go to the loo in the middle of the night. I have a baby alarm in my room. I've forgotten the meaning of independence.

My eyes are tired of straining to see the light in the black tunnel. But, at last, I can see a tiny candle of hope. Something is keeping me going.

A new drug, which has had promising results in America, is going to be tested on guinea-pigs in Bath. I am praying I will get a place on this trial.

I sit in the waiting-room in Bath hospital with my parents, reading the same page of a magazine over and over again. I look at my right hand with its baby-soft skin and long manicured nails painted dark red. But I can't hide the swollen, crooked fingers which serve only as a reminder of this vicious disease I fight each day.

Dad sits in his chair with a pained expression on his face. He has aged. He clutches a newspaper in his hands. 'You must call us if you have a problem, we are here if you need us,' he says tightly.

A nurse hands me the familiar questionnaire, which assesses 'your usual abilities over the past week'.

- *Are you able to dress yourself, including tying shoelaces and doing buttons?*
- *Open a new carton of milk (or soap powder)?*
- *Lift a full cup or glass to your mouth?*
- *Stand up from an armless straight chair?*
- *Run errands and shop?*

And so on . . .

'I find milk cartons a bugger to open!' Mum says, as she watches me ponder whether to tick 'With MUCH difficulty' or 'Unable to do.'

'I can never open them,' Dad adds.

'Darling, you can't even open a can of dog food.'

'I'd love to tick without ANY difficulty to just one of these stupid questions,' I frown, finally ticking 'Unable to do'.

'Sod it,' Dad mutters. It's one of his favourite expressions when he doesn't know what else to say. 'Let's just pray you get on to the trial.'

Mum returns her attention to the *Times* crossword. She gives up, saying she can't concentrate, and reaches down for her knitting. It reminds me of my tennis days and I smile, remembering the cross-country journeys to tournaments and how nervous Mum used to be while watching me play.

'Mum, do you remember that match I played at Eastbourne? And Mrs Betty?! And Peter. I wonder what's happened to them all.'

'What about the time when you were banned from tournament tennis?' she laughs.

'Don't remind me.'

Slowly and painfully I get up from the chair and stretch my legs. I hope my doctor arrives soon. He will be presenting my case in front of the professor who is running the trial. I am feeling anxious.

'Sit down and relax, doctors are always late. What about your first tournament!' she begins, hoping to distract me, her knitting-needles clicking. 'I remember driving you there and you said, "By the way, Mum, I'm going to win this tournament."'

I laugh.

'We didn't know what we were letting ourselves in for, but I did *love* the competitions. I remember your tennis days so vividly.'

Finally, Dr Campbell enters the room. My heart is beating fast. He takes my arm. 'Are you OK?' he asks gently.

'Fine. Nervous,' I smile.

'Good luck,' Mum and Dad say together. Dad's crossing his fingers.

Dr Campbell and I make our way to the conference hall. I take in a deep breath. This could be the beginning of a new life. It may be different. But I want to have another chance . . .

2

The Seed About to Grow

It's 1985. Boris Becker wins Wimbledon this year at the age of seventeen. I am eleven years old.

The school summer holidays have finally begun and all the family are home. Helen, five years older than me, Tom, four years, and Mum and Dad are playing doubles on our neighbour's court. We call them 'lucky pigs' – they have both a tennis court and a swimming-pool. My eldest brother, Andrew, is at home, nervously waiting for A level results.

I am ball-girl, but will be allowed to join in at the end. I hate waiting, I hover impatiently at the side of the court and I want my own, very special racket. I am fed up with being handed the wooden Slazenger which everyone uses.

Tom is having a tantrum, throwing his racket on the ground. Mum and Dad have explained to me that Tom has never been one hundred per cent normal. Born premature, he was a sick baby. At first he nearly died and then his teeth fell out and he had to see a speech therapist.

Tom has terrible mood swings. I don't understand how someone can be happy one minute, sad and angry the next. Dad tells me to keep well out of his way, and not to provoke him until he's calmed down. Which he does, and life carries on as normal again.

'I don't want to play, why should I?' Tom shouts, his weedy figure shuffling around the court.

'I'll play then,' I say, marching towards him.

'No,' he hisses, his blue eyes glaring at me. I back away.

'Tom, give the racket to Alice, let's not have a fight,' Dad says wearily.

'I'll play,' he retorts, holding the racket possessively. 'I've changed my mind.' I hate my brother sometimes. He's mean.

After tennis, Helen and I cycle into town and eat chocolate cake and drink lemonade at our favourite café, Minstrels. Cycling back along Kingsgate Street, I notice a black and gold Pro Kennex racket mounted in the window of a sports shop, priced at £24. I stop and go in, asking the grey-haired sales assistant if I can see it. Picking it up, smelling the leather grip, seeing the silvery strings and the gold and black frame, I know I have to have it. I calculate how long it will take to save the money: with £1.50 pocket-money per week that'll mean sixteen weeks. Too long. I have to earn the money quickly, I think, still holding the racket. Helen's bored and cycles home without me. I have an idea.

My mother runs a second-hand clothes business for children up to the age of twelve from home. It's called 'The Doll's House'. She has over two thousand customers and dresses most of the children in Winchester. She is always busy; piles of clothes need to be priced, labelled, hung up and entered into the system with the owners' names. I go home and ask her how much she will pay me per hour if I help. Mum, surprised by my sudden interest, says, 'Fifty pence.'

Every Wednesday and Friday, the two days she works

in the week, the house is a hive of activity, with mothers buying romper suits and children playing on the landing with an array of toys while Mum tells irate customers that, although the little smocked dress comes from Harrods, she cannot accept it covered with dog hair and with three buttons missing. I love sitting in prime position, writing prices on tags and smiling at customers while folding their clothes and putting them in bags. Mum tells me I am a great help, although she repeatedly has to tell me not to start counting the day's takings while customers are still popping in and out – it is rude. And I must put my chunks of bread, splattered with strawberry jam, on a plate, otherwise messy, sticky crumbs will go everywhere. Rebecca, my next door neighbour and best friend, also helps out to earn extra pocket-money but she gets bored quickly because I never let her sit down; the only thing I allow her to do is hang unwanted clothes back on their rails.

Each weekend I cycle past the sports shop to tell the grey-haired salesman, who is now my great friend, that I will be collecting the racket shortly, and that he must keep one in stock. I go home and write more price tags on almost new salopettes. It won't be too long until the racket is mine.

3

The Elastic Band

October 1985. Andrew is at Surrey University, Helen has gone back to sixth-form boarding school in Marlborough and Tom now goes to a boarding-school for children with learning disabilities. I have finally bought the Pro Kennex racket. All I need now is a smart bag to put it in, a better pair of shoes, a proper water-flask and Ellesse clothes because that's what Chris Evert wears. She is my hero. I'm going to be like her.

Mum and Dad have let me join an eight-week autumn tennis course for beginners at the local recreation ground. The course is held every Saturday morning and the other children are all boys. We have to do warm-up exercises, races bouncing the ball on the racket and the racket frames. Some of the boys cheat, they have Prince rackets with huge heads which makes that exercise so much easier.

'You're OK I suppose, for a girl,' my sulky opponent grunts while shaking my hand. I have just beaten him in the finals of our competition. It was the best of three tie-breaks. I win a mini-sized Mars bar, which I eat in one mouthful, and a tube of bright yellow Slazenger tennis balls.

'Well played, Alice,' the coach says while I am putting my new racket back into its sleeve. 'You show real promise, keep it up.'

I cycle home at top speed to tell Mum and Dad that I won. 'Mum, I'm ready to play you now, I know I am. The coach said I had "true promise" or something like that,' I say, out of breath at the kitchen table.

'Hi, Pudgit,' Dad says, cutting into some cheese. 'Sit down and have some lunch.'

Dad often ignores me. 'Dad. Listen! I'm bored of family doubles. Please can we play, Mum?'

'OK, fine.' She gives in. 'I'll book a court for Monday evening.'

'A proper match?' I ask excitedly.

'Yes, best of three sets.'

Monday morning. I catch the train to school with Rebecca. I go to the Atherley, an all-girls Church of England school. As the train rattles towards Southampton, I wish it was going the other way, back home again. Rebecca and I have double physics first thing, my worst subject. We sit at one of the back tables, talking and making friendship bracelets for each other. During the lesson Mr Wilson, in frustration, throws a piece of chalk at us three times because we are not concentrating. I am looking forward to showing Mum how much I have improved after my tennis lessons and am not in the least bit interested in learning how to wire up a plug.

The match against Mum finally comes. I walk proudly on to the court with my new tennis bag, accessories and racket, pretending I'm at Wimbledon. I am dressed in my marshmallow pink Dash tracksuit and Dunlop Green Flash shoes; my long brown hair is tied neatly into two plaits. I have a white clip which I attach to the back of my tracksuit to hold a ball. Mum tells me I look like a rabbit.

After a few rallies and serves Mum asks, 'Right, are you ready?'

'Yes, ready to beat you,' I chirp happily.

She laughs. 'Rough or smooth, darling?'

The big match begins.

I am quite strong and when I put my weight, which is substantial, behind the ball I can hit it hard. However, Mum is consistently playing the winning shot. I am desperately trying to impress, bobbing up and down, imagining I am Chris Evert. Mum wins the first set and I am irritated that my mother, nearly fifty years old, is beating me.

Half-way through the second set, she double-faults. 'Second serve,' she calls, lining up against the baseline again.

'No, that's game to me, you've had two serves.'

'No, I've only had one.' She then serves two aces, winning the game.

I slam my racket on the ground and hear the frame crack. I look down in fear. I feel sick as I look at the mangled frame. Can I carry on playing, hope Mum won't notice and glue it back together at home? But Mum marches towards me, her face looking as though she is about to explode. She takes one look at the broken racket, snatches her things and starts walking towards the car, proclaiming she'll never play with me again.

I am kicking stones across the pavement. I hate losing but I know I was right. I sit down on a rusty bench and look at my racket. Tears fall on to the broken frame and strings. I want to piece my best friend back together.

Mum buys me a new racket, exactly the same model, but tells me she will not play with a bad sport; I have to learn to control my temper.

The next time we play I tie an elastic band around my wrist. When I hit a bad shot and am about to lose my cool, I flick it hard to stop myself. At the end of the game, my wrist is sore, stripy and red, but at least my racket is still intact and I don't have to walk home.

Mum and I begin to play regularly. As a child and teenager, Mum loved tennis and would have jumped at the chance to play in tournaments and have coaching. She loves sport in general, especially golf. She's pleased that I seem to have found something I really enjoy. She encourages me to play as much as I can. We begin to have a lot of fun together and the games become exciting. Sometimes I beat her and I can see how much she hates losing too. We are two of a kind. I offer her an elastic band.

It's 1986. I am twelve. The summer holidays have come around again quickly. I join an intensive two-week tennis course for young players, run by the same coach I had before, at the recreation ground. On the last Saturday, the coach hands out entry forms for the 'Hampshire County Junior Under Twelve and Fourteen' tournaments. 'When's your birthday, Alice?' he asks me. 'I really think you should enter this.'

'Oh, not until January, January the twenty-fifth.'

'Fantastic, what a lucky birthday, it's obviously fate,' he jokes.

'Why?' I ask, smiling.

'Well, the form asks you to state your age at the end of December in the previous year so you'd only have been eleven, wouldn't you, even though you're twelve now. Someone with a December birthday would have to play in the age group above, although they are only days older than you. See what I mean?'

'Yes, I think so,' I say, dimples in round cheeks reappearing again. He wanders off to talk to another player.

I read the form eagerly. I rush back over to the coach and interrupt his conversation. 'But can I enter this with no results?' I ask, waving the form frantically in front of his nose.

'Everyone has to start somewhere.' He looks amused. 'Go on, give it a go.'

I put the form away in my racket bag and unchain my bicycle. The wheels turn along flat, grey, littered pavements and streets but I feel on top of the world. My first ever tournament.

4

Cheats and Chances

'By the way, I'm going to win this tournament,' I tell Mum in the car.

It's August 1986. Martina Navratilova wins Wimbledon for the seventh time. I am playing in my first County Under Twelve tournament today, at Alverstoke. I put a brand new grip on my racket – bright blue. I have to win. I will win.

Mum and I arrive at Alverstoke. This is terrifying. Now, looking around, I am not so sure I will win after all. 'Be positive, I can win and I will,' I start muttering to myself. 'If I want to win but think I can't, that's negative.'

Boy and girl competitors are practising on the courts, nervous mothers and fathers are talking in the clubhouse. The referee's table is littered with score sheets and match times. I can see a large lady, she must be the Tournament Organizer, standing behind the table with a bright green Penn sweatshirt on, eating a doughnut while opening cans of brand new tennis balls. The draws are pinned to the boards.

One girl stands out among the crowd. She is tall, her dark hair tightly pulled back into a pony-tail, and she's wearing a pink headband which looks like a J-cloth. Her tracksuit is shiny pink to match and her ankle socks even have little pink bobbles on the back too. On her shoulder she carries a bulky silver and red Head racket bag and she is wearing a silver necklace with a tennis racket charm. She looks professional and at least sixteen, not twelve. I wish my navy tracksuit and scuffed trainers could magically transform themselves into something smarter. I do not look like much of a threat.

'Let's go and see who you're drawn against,' Mum says eagerly. She battles her way across the floor, her handbag swinging off her arm, hitting other people. 'This is so exciting. Are you excited, Alice?'

'Mum! Keep your voice down. You're doing it again,' I frown.

'What? Oh look, you're drawn against the number two seed,' she shrieks.

I am playing someone called Imogen Glove. I do not like the name Imogen. It reminds me of a girl I once knew who tied me to a chair and forced me to eat a sand and mud cake.

'What an unlucky draw, oh, bad luck darling,' Mum says in a disappointed tone.

'I haven't lost yet,' I point out indignantly. 'I might win . . . just because she's the number two seed doesn't mean anything.'

'No, of course not,' Mum agrees, eating her words.

I go up to the Tournament Organizer, who is on her second doughnut. There is a big blob of jam on her dimpled chin and little bits of sugar are sticking to her moustache. She looks friendly. She smiles, saying how lovely it is to see a new face. 'Now, love, you're one of the first matches on and I'll be calling out the names any minute now.' She is still opening cans of balls with podgy fingers that look like pork sausages.

I have butterflies in my stomach. What if I lose easily,

what if I do not get a game, a point even? The courts are so open, lots of people can watch. What if I need the loo in the middle of the match? I'd better go now, I think, seeing the 'Ladies' sign across the room. As I am sitting on the loo, my name is called out on the loudspeaker. I feel flustered and sick. I wash my hands, fill my flask with water, my fingers fumbling, and make my way to the referee's table again.

To my horror Miss Bobble Socks is gliding across the room towards the table like an ice skater, her face showing her confidence.

'Imogen, Alice, Court Eight, right at the end. It's the best of three sets and remember tracksuits must only be worn during the warm-up,' the Tournament Organizer says with a beaming smile. She is now eating a huge rock cake.

Our five-minute warm-up is over. I am looking at my flash opponent. Imogen has tested the strings on each of her four rackets and is now changing into her pink and white matching skirt. I am a second-hand Ford Fiesta with stuffing falling out of its holey seats while Imogen is a chic, smooth Jaguar.

'What's your ranking?' she inquires, her nose stuck up in the air. 'I've never seen you before.'

'I don't have one,' I murmur uncomfortably.

'I play on the international circuit, my coach is Swedish,' she says with pride. I look over and see her plastic-looking blond coach smiling at us. I win the toss, electing to receive. She pokes one of the balls into her frilly tennis knickers and struts to the baseline.

Who are those people outside our court? Five chairs are being lined up. A black-haired lady, probably Imogen's mother, is sitting comfortably on a deckchair and it looks like Grandma and Grandpa, with their portable chairs, are watching too. And a young boy. She has brought her whole family along.

Imogen has won the first couple of games. She makes it look so easy, whereas I am scrambling around, scraping balls up, my poor racket frame losing bits of its paint in the process.

First set to Imogen, 6–1. The courts are like school courts, not that that makes any difference – I would still be losing whatever the conditions. But I am sure Imogen hit the last ball, her set point, through the net, not over. Her family clapped too quickly so I did not feel I could question it. Mum has gone back to the clubhouse.

I win the first game of the second set. The worst scenario is to lose 6–1, 6–1, I think. I have won the second game too, and the third. I am beginning to play better. Her mother is pacing up and down behind the netting, she is mouthing something to her daughter. It is my break point to lead 4–1. The ball is coming towards me. It's out! 'Out,' I call.

I hear a shriek. I turn round. Imogen's mother is pinned to the netting, howling like a demented caged animal in the zoo. What is she doing?

'It was in, it was in. You must play two. It landed inside the line,' she screeches. Close up, I can see her crooked teeth and grey hairs.

Imogen is walking up to the net.

'I'm sure it was out,' I exclaim. 'It landed here.' I mark the spot where the ball landed, one foot outside the baseline.

'Oh, no way,' Imogen protests, echoed by her mother. The rest of her family nod in agreement. They look like a judging panel. I want my mum. Where's my mum?

'We'll play two then,' I say shakily, fighting off all the hard stares. I look over to the clubhouse in the distance. There are people wandering about – I should complain. The girl on the next court is crying, she has just run off the court. The referee is dealing with that, I'll just play on. I have double-faulted three times. My chin is wobbling – I think I'm going to cry.

Imogen's mother is challenging all my line calls. She needs glasses. This can't be allowed. I don't know what to do. Why isn't anyone around to see what's going on?

I have lost. My opponent is smiling, shaking my hand as if nothing has happened. Her mother is smiling at me too. Her phoney family are folding up their chairs. If this is what tournament tennis is all about, I have a lot to learn. I am going to find Mum.

'Oh, bad luck, sweetheart,' Mum commiserates before I have even told her I lost. She is drinking a cup of coffee in the clubhouse. She takes another sip. 'I only watched the first set, I found it too nerve-racking. What was the final score?'

'Mum, you must watch next time, you're useless. My opponent was cheating and her mother was a witch.'

Mum comforts me, saying how sorry she is for not having paid enough attention; it will never happen again. 'But there's no need to be downcast, love, you can enter the Plate tournament,' she says, smiling reassuringly.

'The Plate tournament?' I ask hopefully.

'It's the losers' tournament.' She does not know how that sounds – it does not cheer me up. I am a loser. I did not stand up for myself, I let Imogen and her mother walk all over me.

The following morning, Mum and I are setting out for Alverstoke again. I feel much more positive, I have to win one match at least. I am not going home feeling a failure. I am not going home to tell Helen, Andrew, Dad and Tom, especially Tom, that I am out of the losers' tournament. Yesterday, when I told Tom I'd lost, he danced around the kitchen table chanting, 'You wally, you wally.'

My match was scheduled for eleven o'clock. It's now twelve thirty. It has been raining on and off. I wish it would clear up. Mum and I are playing noughts and crosses. I'm going to bring a pack of cards next time, we could play 'shithead', a game Helen taught me.

A mousy boy is hovering on the other side of the clubhouse, waiting to play. The Tournament Organizer calls my match.

'Now if she is who I think she is,' Mum begins, looking at the same boy, who is walking over to the Tournament Organizer, 'I think you have a very good chance darling. I watched her yesterday. She's not very good.'

'Mum!' My elbow nudges her deep in the stomach. 'Will you keep your voice down? Anyway, it's a boy,' I snap. The little boy is standing next to me. He is wearing white shorts and his hair is short and spiky. My opponent can't have arrived yet. The Tournament Organizer hands me the balls. 'You two, Court Five, and try to make it quick, we're running behind already.'

'He's my opponent?' I ask, surprised.

'She is,' the Tournament Organizer corrects me, trying not to laugh. I stare at her again, I can feel myself blushing. I walk quickly out of the clubhouse; the little boy follows me. This time Mum is ready to watch and my opponent's mother and her black labrador, whose leg is in a splint, are also both watching.

I win the first set quite easily. A small, plump lady with curly ginger hair is clapping enthusiastically. She introduces herself to my mother. She looks authoritative, holding a clipboard.

'Who's that?' I ask my opponent eagerly. I am leading 4–1 in the second set.

'She's the County Organizer. Everyone knows her,' she replies, surprised that I've asked.

The County Organizer! I've got to play well now. 'Do you play for the County?' I ask, trying to contain my excitement.

'Yes.'

'He plays for the County, Mum!'

'She, Alice,' Mum says, and then apologizes to the girl's mother.

I could beat a County player and who knows what that might lead to. I imagine shaking my opponent's hand and the County Organizer rushing over to me to ask who I am, saying she simply must have me on her team, she is bowled over by my talent and why hasn't she seen me before? I must impress. Oh no, she is walking away to watch another game. I want to talk to her. Alice, concentrate, you have not won yet. But I can't help dreaming about what it will feel like to hit the last winning shot and win my first match.

I have won. I want to jump in the air, I want to throw my racket into the crowds and throw them my sweaty wristbands. There are only five people watching. Oh well, I still feel happy – I can go home and tell Tom I won. Hooray!

'Well done,' Mum beams with pride. 'It was worth entering this event, you've beaten a County player, you clever girl.'

'What did that woman say?'

'She's the County Organizer . . .'

'I know, I know that. What did she say? Did she say anything about me?'

'She asked me who you were, that's all. She was very nice, quite a funny character.'

I look disappointed. 'Well, what did you want her to say?' Mum asks. I want to know if I'm good enough to play for the County, that's all.

I have reached the FINALS of the Plate Event, beating three County players on the way. I never dreamed I could get this far. Will the bubble burst soon?

Playing on Finals Day gives you an incredible feeling, far removed from the rest of the week. There are professional umpires like at Wimbledon and lots of spectators, players and parents milling around. The table outside is covered with trophies and medals, ready to be picked up and engraved with the winner's name. My greedy eyes are trying to see what I will win. Imogen Glove brushes past me, glancing at the silver trophy with curled handles that she has won two years running. She is in the final of the main event. I really hope the cheat loses.

My final is against Anna, a girl who has been playing in the County for two years. I have got to know her and her parents quite well through the week. They watched one of my earlier matches and congratulated me warmly afterwards. They told me a little about the tennis world, the players and the right tournaments to enter if I'm really serious. Anna's mother has long straight hippy hair which hangs down to her waist. Her father is foreign, small, and has a droopy moustache. He is incredibly keen, passionate even, for his daughter to win, I can see it in his eyes – the tennis scene seems to be his life and joy. Anna is a year younger than me and quite shy. She lets her father do most of the talking although she did ask me whether I liked music – she adores Aha.

We have been called. I am so excited, I can hardly wait.

Anna is a big, strong girl with a long fat plait and chunky thighs. She hits the ball so hard, it is whizzing past me before I can even blink my eye. Mum is talking to her parents. They are laughing, enjoying each other's company.

I am losing, I am not in the same league as this girl. She has won the first set.

I can't believe I've taken Anna to a tie-break in the second set. She looks extremely worried. All the parents have stopped talking. The County Organizer is also watching. I love people watching, it spurs me on.

It's six points to one, match point to her, and I have broken a string in my racket. It is the only one I have. Anna says I can borrow one of hers. It is more powerful. It is 6–5 to her. I think she might take the racket away.

Anna has won 7–5. Her parents congratulate me, saying it could have been anyone's game, we both deserved to win. But it's easy for them to be nice to me, isn't it? Would they have been so nice if I'd won?

The County Organizer is coming up to Anna and me, she's smiling. She puts her freckled arms around us both. 'Well played, well played, you two. Alice, I'm the County Organizer, I run the girls County team.'

'Hello,' I say nervously.

'Anna is a very good player. I've had her in my team for a while now and you mustn't be too disappointed.

She gave you a run for your money, didn't she?' she says, nudging Anna as if she were her favourite pet. 'Alice, have you had any lessons?'

'No, none,' I lie.

Mum gives me a puzzled look. 'You've had a few, Alice.' Mum! I want her to think I'm a natural talent.

'Well, if it's all right with you,' she turns to Mum, 'I'd like to introduce you to Bill Evers, he's the County coach. I'd like to see what he can do with your game. He operates from Winchester.'

'Really? That would be great,' I say, breaking into a huge smile.

She asks me where I come from. We are interrupted by the announcement that the presentation will be held shortly. I collect a small round medal and penholder while enviously eyeing Anna's silver cup. The crowds are clapping, the Tournament Organizer places her large warm hands around mine, telling me I must come back and play next year.

I feel as if I am on a different planet. It might take a while to step back down into the real world again.

'I really want lessons! I want seven lessons a week!' I say in the car, as we drive back home.

'Hang on, Alice. If we're really serious about this, your father and I are going to have to talk about it. Lessons are expensive, we don't have money coming out of our ears.'

'We can afford it though, can't we? We must be able to.'

'We have hefty school fees to pay,' Mum explains. 'It might be a struggle. But come on, it's early days, we need to know what else is involved. By the way, you must ring Granny, she'll be dying to know how you got on today.' Granny is my mother's mother.

Back at home I can hear Andrew's music, 'Waterloo', blasting out of his bedroom upstairs. He still loves Abba. Tom, who is regularly having accidents, has a cut on his forehead and his brown spiky hair is all ruffled.

'Rent! Park Lane with two hotels! Did you win?' Helen asks, looking up. 'Tom, you owe me big time.'

'I give up,' Tom mutters. 'I'm always bankrupt. Look, Alice,' he says proudly, 'I chipped my tooth leap-frogging over a bollard outside the ice-rink.'

I peer into his revolting mouth. 'When did you last clean your teeth?' I say in disgust.

'Shut up. Did you win?'

'No, I lost but I won this.' I flash my penholder at them both.

Helen jumps up and takes my hand, asking me to help her make supper and tell her all about my day. '*Jaws* is on tonight,' she tells me.

Helen, whom I worship, is six foot and towers above me. She was six foot when she was twelve. She is now seventeen and I want to look like her when I'm older – big round blue eyes, high cheekbones and long, thick, dark hair which she tucks behind little ears. I always like it when people say I am a smaller version of her.

'If we watch it, I'll sleep in your room afterwards.'

'Maybe,' she says, 'but you'll keep me up half the night with your sleep talking. You said something about marmalade the other night. So, you played well? Are you going to play in another tournament?'

'Helen!' I exclaim, as if it was the most ridiculous question she could have asked. 'You are looking at . . .' I jump in front of her. 'You are looking at the next Wimbledon champion.'

5

Bill

Two weeks after my first tournament, I rush home after school, fling off my green and gold uniform and quickly dress in my tennis gear. Driving up to the Winchester Tennis and Squash Club, Mum and I see a red sports car parked outside the courts. The County Organizer and Bill Evers are on court five. I join them. I am nervous. This is a chance to be considered for the County Squad.

'Come on, move,' Bill yells impatiently at his pupil. 'No, that's not good enough. You easily had enough time to make that shot. Come on, again.'

I smile at him but he hardly seems to notice.

The County Organizer says, 'He's nearly finished with this girl, he'll be seeing you next. Bill,' she shouts, pointing to her watch, 'you must get on with Alice, it will be dark soon. Come along now.'

'All right, I'll be with you in a minute.' Finally he comes over to us. Bill is tall, has longish hair and is wearing a shiny sea-blue Sergio Tacchini tracksuit.

'This is the young lady I was telling you about, she lost in the finals of the Plate. It was her first tournament,' the County Organizer informs him, standing with her hands on her hips, ready for business. 'She's twelve.'

Bill doesn't appear bothered. Why won't he look at me properly? He shakes my hand half-heartedly, revealing a signet ring and a solid silver chain on one hand. He has an immediate presence. I feel intimidated.

'Let's have a look at you,' he says brusquely. 'Quick, on the baseline.' I run to the other side of the court. We start hitting a few rallies. He looks at my serve. A strand of hair gets in my eyes, I flick it away. 'You need to get a haircut or buy a headband,' he says bluntly, scratching his head and sighing. Only the other day Helen threatened to cut off my long plaits with the kitchen scissors but I want to grow my hair long enough to be able to sit on it. I want to be like my great-great-grandmother who wrote on her passport, under 'distinguishing features', *long hair under knees*. Nervously I throw the ball up to serve again. 'This needs a lot of work,' Bill sighs.

He doesn't like me, he doesn't like me. God! Why didn't you hear my prayer? By the end of the session I am exhausted. My cheeks look like tomatoes.

'You're too fat,' he says. This is totally unexpected, grown-ups aren't supposed to say what they mean. 'How much do you weigh? You need to lose weight.'

At my last school I was teased about being fat; Dad still calls me Pudgit. I am very aware of it. I feel as if I am the odd one out in the family when it comes to 'fatness': Helen is six foot tall and thin; Andrew, who thinks that a helping of ice-cream equals eating the entire box, is unbelievably skinny – I call him 'Hollow legs', and Tom sucks his cheeks in and calls him 'Skeletor'.

'You need to get fit,' Bill hammers on.

The County Organizer shouts, 'Yes, yes, but we can work on that, can't we? Well, what do you think?'

Bill begins picking up the balls with his racket like a magician and aims them into the buckets. I rush to help him, anything to please him. 'Do you want a few more lessons?' he asks me suddenly.

'Yes, definitely, if you have time,' I say humbly, as if speaking to a king on his throne.

'Great, I'll get my diary and we'll fix something up.' He books me in for a lesson after school. 'We'll see how it goes,' he adds, walking off the court. The County Organizer smiles.

I am still frightened of Bill. I'm about to have session number five with him. In the last four lessons we worked hard on my ground strokes, fitness and footwork. I told Bill my favourite player was Chris Evert so we're working on a double-handed backhand like hers.

But I am not sure if he really wants to coach me. He has so many pupils, it is not as if he needs any more. He has told me I have a great deal to improve on. I know that, I just want to show him I am worth coaching.

Bill is firing balls at me from the net. He said 'Last shot' at least twenty shots ago but yet another yellow Dunlop ball flies over the net at the speed of lightning.

'No more,' I pant. 'This is torture, my tummy,' I burst out, surprised by my sudden bravery.

He jumps over the net and walks towards me, a real purpose in his stride. 'Alice,' he says, 'when you are playing at Wimbledon, Centre Court, against Martina Navratilova, are you going to stop the rally saying you've got a stitch?'

'No,' I reply ashamedly.

'No, you're not. Come on, Alicia Peterson Sukova. You can do so much better. You need to be fit, quick, sharp. Fit, quick, sharp,' he says punchily. He runs to the other side of the net and I am trying quickly to pin up my long hair before he hits a ball to me. Bill stares at me again. 'Do you want to do well, be one of the best?'

'Yes.'

'Well, to be a great player, there's just one more thing you need. Please,' he begs, 'get a flipping haircut.'

'It's a sacrifice I must make, think of Bill, tennis,' I am gibbering to take the pain away. I am sitting on the kitchen stool while Mum cuts off my plaits with her proper hair-cutting scissors. She carefully wraps the plaits in tissue and lays them in a drawer in the sitting-room. My head feels so light.

September is over. Lendl wins the US Open. October has started on a major high – Bill has put me into Group D of the County Squad. Group F is the bottom and Group A is the top. Tom and I look at the names and addresses of the twelve players in my group.

'There's a girl called Rosalind who lives at Monkey's Bottom, Filthy Lane,' Tom cackles. 'I'd like to meet her.'

'You're making it up,' I say, snatching the list from him. 'God, you're right!' I smile back at him.

County training takes place at Calshot every other Sunday. Calshot is an activity centre, famous for its sailing, where you can see across the Solent to the Isle of Wight. It's cold, wet and windy. Lining the drive are miserable-looking beach huts that seem to be waiting to be blown down by the gale-force wind.

My session is two hours long. There are four indoor courts and the two back ones are shielded from the dry ski slope by a skimpy curtain. It is no warmer inside. I can see my breath, my hands are purple. Mum says next time she'll wear her red and brown salopettes, snow boots, scarf and ear-muffs.

'Grab a partner and let's hit some balls,' Bill says energetically. Everyone is pairing up around me. I'm scared of being left alone, looking friendless because no one wants me. I spot a tall girl with a blonde pony-tail and ask her to be my partner. Luckily she says yes. We go to one of the back courts. As we are rallying, a skier hurtles down the slope and flies through the gap in the curtain, landing in a heap on my baseline. He doesn't seem hurt.

'Last one to me has to do twenty press-ups,' Bill shouts from the other side of the courts. He is sprinting, and we have to touch him with our rackets. We all run after him in a frenzy, pointing our Slazengers and Wilsons towards him. Rosalind whacks him hard over the head.

While Bill is recovering, holding ice to his head, the County Organizer gives us a pep talk. 'Gather round, gather round – now, girls, six of you will be selected for a County match against Avon next month. We've got a lot of work to do. Whoever's picked,' she leans forward, her eyes out on stalks, 'remember you're playing for Hampshire, for the team, for me.'

'And for yourselves,' Bill adds, winking at me. Bill is definitely taking more notice of me.

It's another Sunday, my fourth time at Calshot, and Mum is driving me there wearing her snowsuit. I love County training, but it's not good enough to be in D, it's not good enough to be the number six player in the Under Fourteen age group. I want to be in the A squad, number

31

one. Their sessions are three hours long, I want to practise with the better players – I feel I have so little time to get good.

I can't wait to see Bill and talk about the results of the County match against Avon last Sunday. We had to wear County tracksuits for the day. They were silver and red, with 'Unigate' (who sponsor us) stamped on the jackets. I was last on the list, number six. I had to play two singles matches against Avon's number five and number six players. Then doubles with Emma, the girl with the blonde pony-tail. I lost one match but beat the number six and Bill was watching all the time. He said I'd be picked for the next match against Sussex, which is soon. I'm beginning to think he likes me, really likes me. Through Bill, I am learning so much about the tennis world. As well as County matches, he tells me the tournaments to enter throughout the year to get results. We've made a list:

1 Winchester Open – international players
2 Surbiton
3 Pit Farm
4 Solihull
5 Alverstoke
6 Nationals at Edinburgh and Eastbourne – although unlikely I'll get in next year.

A new world is opening up in front of my eyes.

6

The Regional Trial

It's January 1987. Navratilova loses to Hana Mandlikova in the Australian Open. I have made a chart of where I want to go in tennis.

Step One   County = Hampshire and the Isle of
                 Wight – Number One.
Step Two   Regional. South Region = Players from
                 Hampshire, Berkshire, Buckinghamshire
                 and Oxfordshire – Number One.
Step Three National standard = Being one of the
                 best players in the country. National
                 Tournaments – Edinburgh, Eastbourne,
                 Bournemouth, Wimbledon. Need
                 results to get into these tournaments.
                 Need to beat other national players.
Step Four International tournaments
Step Five Wimbledon, Grand Slams! Be number
                 one in the WORLD.

I haven't shown anyone my journey yet, they might laugh. But I've made a start, I have lost a lot of weight. My diet has changed – white bread has turned to brown, chocolate and crisps have been replaced by yoghurts and fruit, and each night I do press-ups, sit-ups and skipping in my bedroom. Dad says it sounds as if I'm going to come crashing down through the floorboards. I also go running after school. It is dark in the evenings, so Mum takes the car and I run alongside her; Mum times me and I keep a record of the times in my fitness diary. Rebecca, my best friend, and I go swimming after school too, although I don't know how long that will last. We both get bored too quickly just swimming up and down, up and down.

I'm in Group C at Calshot and because of my County match results I have been selected for a South Regional Trial in February. I hardly dare imagine what would happen if I was accepted into the Region – the most terrifying and most exciting thing I've ever had to think about.

We all talked to Bill over Christmas about my tennis. Bill said he had 'great plans for me'. But then there was the money side of things. Holding his hand on his chin, he said he knew how expensive it was, and that it would only get more expensive if I got into the South Region. I stopped breathing. We had to be able to afford lessons.

'I would like to coach Alice twice a week to prepare her for the Regional Trial. But it's not only lessons. It's rackets, shoes, petrol for travelling, tournament fees, bed and breakfasts, restringing, clothes, so many things. It is hard,' Bill confessed.

'And it's the time, Alice. Not only yours but ours,' Dad said seriously, stroking his grey hair into place.

Bill looked at Mum. 'All I can say is that this girl has a huge talent and given the chance, she could make it to the top.'

I adore him! Restraining myself from hugging Bill, I looked over to my parents, my head dizzy with dreams of the future. Dad still looked serious. He is a thinker, he digests information before you can detect any kind of reaction. His caution annoyed me but I could see the immediate glow in Mum's eyes. She is ambitious for me. She broke the silence. 'My money from the business can be put towards it. I would have loved this chance, Alice must have it.'

Dad nodded in agreement. 'If this is what you really want, Alice, we'll support you all the way,' he said, eventually breaking into a smile, his gold tooth shining.

Bill thanked my parents. 'You won't regret it, she's got a great career ahead of her. I'll see you on the court tomorrow, kiddo, five o'clock. Don't get too big-headed now, we've got a lot of work ahead of us.' He put his hand on my shoulder for a moment and then left.

Peter Hamilton, the South Region coach, is dividing us into groups, giving us various hitting exercises to do. It is the day of the trial. Peter has dark curly hair and a trim moustache. How can someone so small look so severe?

'Hey, you, Reebok top, what's your name?' he asks, pointing to me.

'Alice.'

'Right, team up with Connie. I want you to do the drilling exercise forehand down the line. Go.'

Peter marches from one court to another with his clipboard. He ought to be in army uniform. Why hasn't he been near me yet? I've just hit a winner. Why couldn't he have been watching? Connie hits a winner past me. I turn around and he is standing right behind me. 'Come on, wake up,' he orders fiercely, although I feel as if his eyes are laughing at me. 'Here's a ball. Let's see you hit some more, and tie that lace up before you fall flat on your face.'

'You're not bad, the lot of you,' Peter says at the end

of the trial. 'I'll be writing to you in the next ten days or so. Remember if you're not picked this time, maybe next. Go on, off with you,' he smiles.

Please choose me.

I have two letters. One from Helen, the other from Peter. Which first? Helen's. It is Helen's gap year and she's in Australia, travelling, picking grapes for six months. I miss her.

'Al, I'm starving. I'm working so hard and eating loads of peanut butter on toast to keep me going. I'm also drinking lots of delicious wine. You would love it out here. How's the tennis going?'

Sorry Helen. I have to know. I put down the half-read letter and rip open the other.

'. . . could I emphasize that this invitation does not mean that your place is guaranteed in the Squad throughout the year, for if appropriate standards of behaviour and attitude on and off the court are not maintained, your place will be in jeopardy. Failure to do the following could also mean exclusion from the squad:

1. To enter the appropriate National age group championships.

2. To submit when requested your tournament results for ranking purposes.

'Bill, I've got in, I've got in. The letter came this morning,' I shriek down the phone.

7

Training

It's May 1987. I'm at school in a double French lesson, clock-watching. Straight after the bell rings I'm going to a South Region residential weekend at Halton.

Over the last three months every weekend has been taken up with tennis – regional tournaments, six-hour training sessions, inter-regional tournaments, residential weekends and tournaments against schools. Mum and I live in the car, clocking up the mileage.

Occasionally I feel different from my schoolfriends. They go clothes shopping, go to sleepovers, go to the cinema at the weekends. They are also beginning to go out with boys, have crushes, snog after school or in lunch breaks. Conversations revolve around who likes who. Sometimes I wish I had more free time to be normal and go to their parties. I am interested in boys, although I can't see myself going out with anyone yet. I love what I'm doing. Rebecca cannot believe I don't get bored. But I don't – I am so happy.

'Who's going to be at this weekend?' Mum asks as we drive to Halton.

'Hopefully, Connie,' I reply. I have become good friends with Connie. She plays in the same regional group as me and is also my doubles partner. We're like twins on court: the same height (five foot five), light brown hair, freckles splattered over our noses. I stayed with her during a tournament in the Easter holidays. We won a doubles event, winning £5 each which we spent at Fenwick. I bought some socks, blue with little sheep on them, and Connie bought a freckle-removing cream. Connie's mother is Irish, small, slim and pretty – she reminds me of Felicity Kendal. She sells tropical plants. She always seemed to be handling the prickly plants with her rubber gloves and packing them into her little white van. She gave me an exotic plant to take home, which Mum put in the loo. Connie's father is a construction engineer who also has a racket-stringing business. This is useful as I am constantly breaking strings.

'Anna will probably be there too,' I say.

Anna was the girl with the long plait and chunky thighs whom I played against the year before at Alverstoke. As a baby she played with a mini tennis ball in her cot. Instead of having the usual toys and dolls her father hung a ball on a string which she would hit endlessly up and down. Her parents are desperate for her to be successful and so she's pushed hard. At the last regional tournament I saw her father hiding behind the curtains framing the court whispering, 'Play on her forehand, attack her weak serve.' She won and he placed a nugget of gold in her hand. I'm quite envious. I asked Mum if I could have £1 whenever I won. She said no.

'What do you enjoy most about these weekends?' Mum asks.

'I can tell you what I hate most,' I reply, 'the fitness exercises and the dreaded running machine! It always seems to make an appearance at the end of the weekend, when we're all tired.'

'Sounds awful,' Mum laughs.

'It bleeps and in between the bleeps, which become quicker and quicker, you have to run a certain distance, I dread dropping out first. I hate running too, Peter loves to drag us across fields in the morning. We have to get up at seven-thirty, it's so early!'

I flip the little mirror down in the front seat of the car. 'Do you think we look like each other, Mum?' I ask, changing the subject.

'Well, we've both got quite thin faces, blue eyes, small nose . . . you don't have my long chin though, or my curly hair. You're much fairer than me. Damn, I think we've missed the turning.'

'I've got Dad's big ears. I'd rather have your little ears. And I've got his teeth. My brace is killing me, I just want to pull it off,' I frown, tugging at the metal in frustration.

'We never had orthodontists in our time, so look how mine turned out.' Mum turns to show me her mouth of crooked teeth. 'Now concentrate, Alice, was that the last turning to Halton?'

Finally we arrive at Halton. The place is like a community centre. The bedrooms are in blocks outside the main building.

'Have a lovely time,' Mum says too loudly. 'I'll be here to pick you up . . .'

I kiss her quickly and push her back into the car. It's not cool to hug your mum for too long.

I collect the key to my room, throw my bags on to my bed and then meet everyone in the main common-room. We are a group of eight. I sit down at the round table next to Connie. There is a pool table on the other side.

'We're sharing together,' Connie whispers.

Peter is dressed in his red and blue Slazenger tracksuit,

armed with paperwork. 'Alice, hi,' he says. 'Can you hand round the weekend schedules?' I look down at the sheets. The theme for the weekend is, 'The mental side of the game and positive self talk'. 'Believing in yourself is the key,' Peter tells us. 'The mental side is just as important in the game. Tennis is like a jigsaw puzzle, one piece missing and the whole picture is ruined.'

Connie is not paying attention, scribbling a note to me saying how much she fancies Jason sitting opposite her. I write back saying I prefer Luke. I feel an arm over my shoulder.

'You're not here for fun,' Peter reminds us, taking the piece of paper from me. 'Don't think that for a second.' His eyes skim the note before chucking it in the bin. 'You're here to play tennis,' he reminds us. 'Anyone who fools around will be out.'

After a rundown about the weekend's timetable, we have some free time. We eat supper in the canteen and then play pool.

It's Saturday afternoon. My legs feel wobbly from the strenuous fitness exercises we did all morning. I'm glad finally to be on court. Peter and the other regional coach are working on player reports. They assess our general technique, physical movement, mental attitude and how much effort we put into the sessions. I need my report to be good. I moved up recently from the E group to the C group, but I must get into the A group. We are on court for five hours.

In the evening, we watch part of the famous 1980 Wimbledon final, Borg v. McEnroe.

'Borg first became interested in tennis as a child; his father gave him a racket which he had won in a ping-pong tournament,' Peter begins. 'He left school when he was fourteen and within a year became the world's top class junior player . . .'

Fourteen. I could leave school in a year.

'He's a true inspiration to us all. His temperament is wonderful,' Peter carries on, sliding the video the wrong way into the machine. One of the boys jumps up and does it for him. Peter laughs, saying he cannot work his own video recorder, let alone other people's.

It is a marathon match which Borg wins eight games to six in the final set. I am mesmerized. He never gives up or loses his head. I am going to do the essay Peter has set us on Borg.

It's Sunday morning, and Connie and I are tucking into a big breakfast of greasy bacon, eggs and toast. The early morning run through the mud and across the fields is thankfully over. Feeling bloated, we make our way to the courts, where we find Peter bouncing up and down on his feet, ready to kick off the session.

On court, I know I have to perform well as it's match play today. There's a boy called Tim Henman whom I'd like to play against, as I find I play much better against really good players.

'. . . but first of all let's warm up. Alice, go with Tim, Connie with Jason . . .' Connie's eyes light up, her cheeks go pink.

Later, I play a match against Anna which I win in two straight sets. It is the first time I have beaten her, surprising both Peter and myself.

'Well done. I've been impressed by all of you on and off the court,' Peter says at the end of the weekend, genuinely pleased. 'Remember, essays in next week and we'll be sending your player reports shortly. Oh, and before you leave,' Peter says with a wry smile, 'there's just one more exercise we haven't done.'

The running-machine, how could I forget?

8

A Day in the Life of a Tournament . . .

Finals Day. 'This is the third and final announcement for Alice Peterson. Could she please come to the desk. We want to begin the match. Her opponent is waiting. Spectators are waiting for you,' says the Tournament Organizer crossly.

'I'm so sorry.' Mum sways. 'I can't think where she is.' Mum's drunk. She always has one glass of wine but I think the pressure of Finals Day is just too much.

'She'll be disqualified,' warns the Tournament Organizer.

My feet won't move. They want to, but they just won't. I'm so nervous.

I hear the announcement. 'She's disqualified, disqualified . . .'

'No!' I scream, sitting up in bed. I look around. My clothes are still neatly folded on my chair. Thank God. I made a list last night of the favourite things I'd wear for finals:

1 New shirt with little coloured triangles on arms.
2 Navy tracksuit.
3 White plaited headband.
4 White Ellesse socks with red bobbles on back
  (I love Ellesse clothes but Mum says they are a rip off – can afford socks though).

5 New Reebok trainers.
6 Granny knickers so I can put ball into them –
  having to borrow Mum's.

I jump out of bed and get dressed.

Breakfast time.

'Remember to fill your water-flask with fresh water,' Mum nags. 'One girl got terrible diarrhoea because her water was a week old.'

Tom finds this insanely funny and spills his tea to join the tomato ketchup stains on his jumper. He pulls a silly face at me.

'Granny wants to come and watch you today too. We'll take one of the fold-up chairs.' Granny is doing what she calls her 'royal tour' of all her children. She comes into the kitchen and kisses both Tom and me good morning, then sits down to eat her orange, cut into neat segments, and her piece of bread with honey. Granny is eighty-six and remarkably fit. The only thing beginning to fail is her eyesight. She's wearing a pretty pale pink shirt, clasped with a round silver brooch.

'We used to have terrific tennis parties out in Africa,' she says nostalgically. Granny's life is full of contrast and change. She was brought up at Longford Castle, near Salisbury in Wiltshire, but made a life for herself out in Africa in the 1920s and 30s. She and Grandpa created a farm and a home from untamed African veldt in Rhodesia. Mum longs to return to see her old home, where she spent the first ten very happy years of her life. I'd like to go too. Maybe I will some day.

'Your grandpa made a court out of antheap soil. We

44

used to play in the cool of the evening, when the farm work was over for the day.'

'Were you any good, Granny?'

'Well, I was quite,' she nods.

'Will you be ready to leave in ten minutes?' Mum asks.

'Yeah, ready now really.'

'You and Mum are always disappearing. Leave me behind, I don't care,' Tom says as he slams his spoon into his cereal bowl. Milk spills over the tablecloth.

'Tom, we've talked about this,' Mum reminds him wearily. 'You must not get jealous. Your father's taking you out to play golf today, isn't he?'

'That's right,' Granny says sternly.

'Um,' he mutters indifferently, shrugging his shoulders. 'Don't know, don't care. It's all about Alice, isn't it?' he snarls. 'Never me.'

'Tom, shut up,' I order. 'You're seventeen, not seven.'

'Alice! Please, what are you doing?' Mum asks incredulously. 'You've had all morning to get ready. Come on.' However much time I leave, I am always late.

On our way to the tournament in Guildford, the warmth of the car and Mum's classical music make me fall asleep instantly. Mum has to poke and prod me with the steering-wheel lock fifteen minutes before we arrive. 'Wake up, darling, you mustn't be lethargic when we arrive.'

We finally reach the club. 'Ma, we're here, wake up,' Mum says, trying to arouse the second sleepy passenger. 'Did I put sleeping pills in your coffee this morning?' she asks, smiling.

'Wide awake, darling, I haven't been asleep at all,'

Granny says, immediately opening her eyes. 'Very well driven.'

No time to think about Granny's uncanny ability not to be asleep even though her mouth was open, her eyes were shut, and she treated Mum and me to the occasional snore. I have to get my brain into tennis mode. Start thinking about winning.

The matches are running two hours late because of the rain. Players and parents are huddled in the clubhouse, a muddle of see-through anoraks and hoods, eating egg rolls and Twix bars and looking miserable. Moans and groans about the weather and the hanging around are flowing from every corner of the room. Granny is staring vacantly into space, her chin is stuck out and she is sliding her false teeth around, a habit she is totally unaware of. I must stop her doing that, I think desperately.

'Granny?'

'Yes, darling?' she says, immediately alert. False teeth are kicked back into their correct position.

'I'm bored. Tell me a story about your time in Africa.'

Granny has so many stories, she has to think about it for a moment. 'Well,' she says at last, 'I'm sure Mum has told you about the time when we went riding and a black mamba reared its ugly head in front of our horses. And your uncle saved us, shooting its head off. I'll always remember the image of him cycling home, the body of the snake wrapped round his bicycle.'

'Ugh,' I cringe. 'Tell me another . . .'

'Oh, hello, Alice,' Mrs Betty chirps, interrupting us with her high-pitched voice, sticking her tongue out. 'My Julie did so well in this tournament three years ago.' She looks momentarily crestfallen. Then she perks up,

'What time are you playing, I'd love to watch your match.' Tongue pokes out and eyes sparkle again.

Everybody knows Mrs Betty. Her daughter gave up but she continues trailing around the tournaments throughout the year, her little granny bag hanging off her arm. The tennis scene was so much part of her lifestyle and her routine that she found it impossible to give up.

Finally, I am called. I have the butterflies, my stomach feels as if it's permanently going over a humpback bridge at full speed.

While I'm playing, Mum has to do something with her hands. She always brings her knitting along and is currently making a brown Jaeger jumper for Helen. A glass of wine sits at her feet. A Hampshire mother who reeks of scent settles down next to her. She is wearing a chic, shoulder-padded Joan Collins type outfit, and holds two very well-groomed Yorkshire terriers. Mum cringes at the sight of the red bows in their hair and the little tartan rugs over their backs.

'What sweet little dogs,' Mum coos. 'How did your daughter do in her final?'

'She lost.'

'Oh, I'm sorry, she – ' Mum is cut off.

'Oh, but she did not sleep at all well last night,' the other mother adds quickly. 'We live above a pizza restaurant and it gets quite rowdy on a Friday night. She would have won if she hadn't been so tired, poor love. How's Alice doing?'

'I'm not sure. I think she's winning.' Mum tries to sound casual. She actually knows the score down to the last point. I am one set up, two games all, deuce. Mums in general like to pretend they're not paying attention.

The match is very tight. One set all, four games all. I am fighting for every point. Mum is pulling her knitting apart, the wool strewn everywhere. Granny howls with laughter whenever I miss an easy shot but really I don't think she can see the ball too clearly. She sometimes calls out 'Bad luck' when I've hit a winner. I can hear Mum trying to hush her, telling her that it was OK: 'It was in, Mummy, that's Alice's game,' she whispers loudly.

'Oh!' Granny cackles. 'Jolly good.'

I have won! After a sweaty handshake, I turn round and can see Mum and Granny clapping vigorously.

'Clever girl.' Granny congratulates me over and over again.

Mrs Betty is clapping too. I feel as if I have reached the top of a mountain nobody told me I'd ever be able to climb. I have done it.

We wait until the end of the day for the presentation.

'And the winner of the Girls Under Fourteen Tournament, Alice Peterson.' There is more clapping. I climb up the wooden steps to collect my cup and a brown envelope with £20. I could buy half an Ellesse top with that.

At home, I'm in bed, my silver trophy lying next to me. I'm going to get it engraved tomorrow. Because of my lucky January birthday, I have one more year in the Under Fourteen age group after this summer. I pray that this tournament is my passport into the Under Fourteen Nationals for next year.

9

Edinburgh

I am fourteen. It's March 1988. It's two months until the Nationals at Edinburgh. I am waiting for the letter with the acceptance list. I have to be accepted, I want Bill to be proud of me.

'Alice, I think the letter's finally come,' Mum shouts from the bottom of the stairs.

I rush down. The envelope has the LTA stamp on it. I rip it open. There are typed names in alphabetical order but mine isn't there. Mine isn't there. I can't believe it, I should be playing. I feel a lump in my throat. 'Well, I didn't get in again, Mum, I am not even on the reserve list.' I swallow hard, pushing the piece of paper in her direction, feeling tears burn my eyes.

Mum scans the list. She flicks the sheet over – Cross, K.M. (Karen), Donovan, K.M. (Kelly), Metcalfe, M.L. (Melissa), Peterson A.D. (Alice), Pullin, J.M. (Julie) . . . Disappointed lips widen, eyes light up. 'You are looking at the wrong side, you silly girl. That's the Under Twelve age group. Look, see,' she corrects me, pointing at my name.

I seize the lists back from her. I can see names I recognize.

Peterson A.D. (Alice). Relief. Happiness. Tears smudge my name. Connie's name is there too. I rush back upstairs to my bedroom and, like a teacher with a red pen, tick a

49

big tick next to Step Three on my chart. Now I've just got to practise, practise and practise . . .

I am in Edinburgh on a Saturday evening, squashed in the back seat of the South Region minibus, tennis racket bags, tapes, sweets and ice-cream wrappers, bottles of water and more clobber at my feet. Peter is driving, following the large yellow AA signs to the 'Junior National Tennis'.

'Look, Junior Nationals,' I say, nudging Connie who is half asleep. She takes off her Walkman. I feel excited – the bright yellow signs make me feel like a serious tennis player, almost a star.

I have never ventured so far north. Bright lights skirt the streets, doors are opened to clubs and restaurants. It seems lively and friendly. Connie and I are pointing out places we want to go to. I want to explore, I want to win, I want to eat, I want to see what our hotel's like. My stomach is knotted up with nerves.

Sunday comes, the day before the tournament begins, and I am practising on the hard courts with Peter and the rest of the Region. The venue is impressive, the courts are kept in good condition. Centre Court, singled out on its own, is like a shrine. I feel overwhelmed by the whole event; watching a few of the other National players, the standard is much higher than ordinary tournaments. I am ranked number three or four in the Region Under Fourteen and I'm number two in the County, I've had good results. Yet fear of embarrassment, doubt, little faith in myself and images of losing 6–0, 6–0 start to creep into my mind. These negative thoughts are buzzing around my mind like mosquitoes. I need to zap them. Peter tells us 'he wants results', but quickly mutters, his head down, 'But all you can do is go out there and play your best.'

Coaches, players, parents are all milling around in nervous anticipation. Peter is definitely on edge, hoping one of his six players makes a mark.

There is a players' meeting at six o'clock. The room is crowded. Players from all over the country are competing – Devon, South Wales, Cambridge, Somerset, Essex, Durham. I recognize a few people but I am sitting with Connie, sticking close to a familiar face. The Director is going over the rules; the Championship Secretary is crossing off the competitors' names.

'Phil Mycock.' Everyone laughs.

'Alice Peterson.'

'Yes,' I squeak, and then have a coughing fit. Connie thumps my back. 'Choke up chicken,' she whispers. I had rehearsed my 'Yes' all through the meeting and it still came out wrong.

We turn the pages of the programme to see the Under Fourteen draw. It is a draw of sixty-four; the names of the eight seeded players are written in bold capitals. My name is under capitals.

'I am playing the number four seed,' I say to Connie in disbelief.

'I'm playing the number three seed. Well, this will be a quick tournament,' Connie predicts dryly, closing the programme as if to say, 'Well, that's it, the END, draw the curtains.' 'Who are you umpiring?' she asks.

'Oh no, I am umpiring on Number One Court.' Number One Court would have to be one of the most conspicuous courts. We both laugh. I don't know whether I'm happy or sad with my draw.

'This is a joke,' Connie smirks. 'First Nationals and we get draws like this. We've got no chance.'

'Come on, so what,' I stress, grinning back. 'We can win, Connie.'

It is Monday and the first morning of the Nationals. Everyone is huddled around Centre Court, waiting for the introduction ceremony. It is bitterly cold, a howling gale is blowing around us and tartan rugs are on virtually every mother's lap.

'How was your night, Mum?' I ask, shivering. Mum is staying with friends.

'The bed was rock solid, like sleeping on the floor and . . .'

Mum's night is soon forgotten as men in kilts walk down the steps, playing bagpipes. Suddenly, I feel really lucky to be here; whether I win or lose, I have made it to the Nationals and I feel proud. This is a wonderful experience, I wouldn't change it for the world. Who knows, I might win today. I'm beginning to feel really excited. The first matches are called.

I am wandering around, watching a few of the matches. Tim Henman is playing on Centre Court. I watch him for a while. On another court I hear shouting. 'Play two?! The ball was miles out. What a crap call . . .' I love watching arguments. A referee is talking to the player, giving her a warning. Umpiring is far more nerve-racking than playing. Oh God, I need the loo again.

My name has been called – I am umpiring Karen Cross v. Tamsin Wainwright. I hope it is a quick match. The three of us are walking to the court, Karen striding ahead. I'm climbing on to the high chair, my legs are wobbling. The height of embarrassment would be to fall off before

I have even reached the top. Thank goodness, I am now sitting, the scoresheet on my lap, trying to look casual, as if everything is under control.

The five-minute warm-up is over. The match starts. 'Miss Cross won the toss and elected to serve,' I say, my voice wavering. I'm twisting the pencil around in my fingers.

I have to pencil in every point played. It's gone to three sets. So far I've had only a few filthy stares from the players when they thought I'd called incorrectly. Come on, one of you hurry up and win, I don't care who.

The match is over, everyone's clapping. The winner beams at me. I feel as if I have won too. I'm so relieved it's all over. Now I can concentrate on my match.

It is four o'clock and I've been called. Connie has just lost and looks miserable. She gets so angry with herself if she plays badly. She comes up to me and shrugs. I give her a hug. She manages a 'Good luck, play better than me,' and quickly goes off to avoid confrontation with Peter. She can't face him quite yet. My opponent towers above me, she looks as if she does body-building. The player whom I umpired this morning is umpiring me. She is in a good mood because she won. She seems to know my opponent well, they are laughing, standing close together.

On Number One Court, my legs are shaking like jelly. I can't get a rally going. I want to win so much, but I am almost scared to. My opponent is ranked number four in the country under fourteen. People are watching. This is daunting, terrifying, exciting. I must play well. I can win, I can win. You will win, Alice. Positive self-talk. The five minutes is up and I'm changing into my skirt. It is still cold but those are the rules. I suddenly try to remember what colour knickers I'm wearing because the wind is blowing so hard it's giving everyone a good look now and then. My opponent is glugging down some water. She quickly pins her blonde hair back off her face, picks up a couple of balls and walks to the baseline. She walks with the confidence of a super-model. She wins the toss and starts to serve.

LOVE FIFTEEN, LOVE THIRTY, LOVE FORTY . . . nothing is going over the net. The balls are all on my side. I love the net. Mum's face crinkles up as I hit another shot into the bottom of the net . . . GAME.

She has lobbed me. I am running backwards, I've lost my footing. I am flat on the ground. My elbow hurts, I've scraped a layer of skin off my knee. It's raw and red. Ouch, it stings.

'Are you OK?' my opponent asks.

I get up quickly. 'Yes, fine.' I battle on.

GAME, GAME, GAME.

'Miss Hamplett leads five games to love,' the umpire says. Ssh! Do you have to say it so loudly? I think, in a mood of despair.

Defeated. Months of practising and it is over in under an hour. Bitter disappointment. I've let myself down, let Bill down. My friends at home, Helen, Tom and Andrew will all see the results in the newspaper tomorrow. I can see Mum folding up her portable chair. Peter is twitching and hovering around. My opponent waits for me, we walk off court together. Time to face disappointed friends.

If only I could rewind and start all over again. I could have won.

10

Fractured Nerves

It's August 1988: Stefan Edberg and Steffi Graf are the
Wimbledon champions this year and watching them kiss
their trophies on Centre Court makes me want to be
there. I went up on the second Tuesday, to Number One
Court, but it rained all afternoon and I was sitting next
to a man who had terrible BO.

I'm at Devonshire Park, Eastbourne, playing in the Under
Fourteen Nationals. This is the equivalent to the Nation-
als at Edinburgh, but whereas Edinburgh was played on
hard courts, this is the Prudential Junior *Grass* Court
Championships of Great Britain. It's Wednesday, Day
Three of the tournament.

The sun is shining. The grass courts still look immacu-
late, the white painted lines shining. I love this venue.
Professionals have played here, there is a wonderful
atmosphere. There is certainly something special about
playing on grass because Wimbledon is played on this
surface.

A few old people are settling down on their stripy
deckchairs to watch more of the tennis. They are sucking
syrupy sweets. One says, 'I love watching the youngsters,
I come every day, it's such a treat.'

In the evenings Connie and I go to the pier and play
on the fruit-machines. The beach is at our doorstep. The

sounds of seagulls fill the salty sea air. I almost feel I'm on holiday.

I won my first two rounds and I'm playing the number four seed again, the same girl that I lost to in Edinburgh. I'm longing to play her again. I'm a different player from how I was in Edinburgh – more confident, stronger mentally. I'm not scared of winning. Bill believes in me, and I'm beginning to believe in me too. I know my opponent thinks she'll win, I overheard her saying what an easy draw she had, that she had another 'walkover match' today against me. She didn't see me, but Connie and I were right behind her. Connie wanted to say something but I put my hand over her mouth before she could.

If I win, I'll be in the quarter-finals. I'll be an unknown in the last eight. I wish Bill was here to support me but Helen's here instead, just back from the Edinburgh Festival, where she's been acting in a play. I think she's more excited than me. She keeps poking and prodding me, asking me when I'm playing. Whenever anyone vaguely good-looking walks past, she asks me whether I fancy him. She's never watched me before in a proper tournament. I hope she behaves.

'You've been called Ali, go, go,' Helen squeaks. 'Good luck,' she says, hugging Mum in excitement. 'You can do it.' Her big floppy hat blows in the wind.

Anna is umpiring me. I have lost the first game to love. Changeover. My opponent looks too content.

A big round o sits next to my name on the scoreboard; 3 is next to Sara's – she looks so relaxed she might as well be asleep.

I have won a point. I have won a game. She's lost her

concentration. I have won four games in a row. Helen is jumping off her seat and clapping loudly, in contrast to Mum who sits quietly on her chair, trying to hide her excitement. I smile at both of them at the changeover. I am leading, four games to three.

'Right, come on, this is your chance, beat this girl, make her run a bit more,' I mutter to myself. 'She's not that good.' My right thigh looks red from where I've been slapping it, saying 'Come on' after each point and each game.

Mum is darning Tom's socks but I know her beady eyes have not missed a point. Helen tugs on her sleeve when I miss an easy shot. Her dungaree strap has fallen off her arm, her hat fell off ages ago.

I serve an ace. 'First set to Miss Peterson, six games to three,' Anna says. My opponent slumps in her chair like a heavy bag of potatoes and throws her racket down.

I'm losing the second set. I've got to keep telling myself I can win. Forget she's a seed. You can win.

One set all. My opponent looks calm again. Many people have gathered round the court. Anna's parents are watching, along with Connie who has been watching most of the time. Occasionally we catch each other's eye and her smile is saying, 'I never thought you could do it, but come on!' Peter is watching, his clipboard still stuck to him.

Five all in the final set, deuce. I have hit a winner, people are clapping. I feel as if I'm on television. My opponent's screaming. Great, she's rattled. Mum can barely watch, her sewing's been abandoned, she's trying to look calm but I can tell her emotions are flying. She is twisting her pearl studs around, grinding them into her earlobe. Helen is shifting up and down on her seat as if she has something up her bottom. Her long wavy hair looks wild. As I'm serving they both clench their fists, terrified I'll do a double fault and let go of my advantage. The serve is in – they put their faces in their hands when the ball flies out. Back to deuce.

MATCH POINT to me. Just one more point, that's all I need, one tiny little point. The rally is long. Hit it in the net, in the net, I think. 'Hit it out, out,' Mum is saying vigorously under her breath, while Helen is murmuring, 'Miss it, go on, miss it.' She hits a forehand, it lands on the inside tramline. I hit a backhand cross court. It's too short. She hits a backhand approach shot into the middle of the court and charges to the net. She is at the net, all I need to do is pass her – I have the whole court. I've hit it past her. The crowds gasp. It is inches out. Mum looks as if she is on the top of a cliff, dangling at the edge – every point I miss makes her fall, it is painful. Helen is beside herself, she can't watch any more. She's bent over in her chair, legs tightly crossed, head down, as if she's suffering from chronic indigestion.

Second match point. She hits a ball that is definitely out. I look at Anna, desperately waiting for her to call, 'Game, set and match.' Instead she calls, 'Deuce.' What a time to make such a terrible line call. Keep your cool, do not lose your concentration now.

Third match point. Another long rally. She hits a drop shot. I run to the net and scoop it up. It's a weak shot but at least I got it back. She smashes a forehand right into my body. She wants to kill me. Quick reflex. I stick my racket out and hope for the best. I hit a volley which clips the net, wobbles . . . everything is on pause for a couple of seconds. It lands on her side of the court. My

58

opponent grunts in pain. I have won the match! Helen cries, jumping up and down and clapping her hands until the palms are burning the colour of red chillies. She accidentally knocks the old man sitting next to her, his peardrop dribbles out of his mouth. After two and a half hours it is over. I rush to the net, get a sloppy handshake, no eye contact, and shake Anna's hand. 'Well done!' she says, 'I'm so stiff from sitting all that time!' I put my rackets away. I'm shaking. I want to ring Bill and tell him I am in the quarter-finals; my thoughts are racing. I can see my opponent is in tears as she trails off the court.

People congratulate me, people I don't even know. Mum hugs me so tightly I think I'm going to be squeezed to death. 'I knew you could do it – I am so proud of you,' she says. Happy tears flow down her sun-tanned cheeks. She finally lets go and breathes deeply. 'You held your nerve beautifully. That was agony, I was more nervous than you.'

'I feel as if I've been playing too, I'm exhausted,' Helen yawns, putting her hand, sweaty with heat and nerves, around my shoulder. 'I don't know how Mum can watch you all the time, my nerves are fractured! I'll get varicose veins from crossing my legs so much. I need a drink after that, is there a bar here?' I laugh and snatch her hand excitedly, pulling her off to get a drink.

The old man who lost his boiled sweet limps towards me. 'Well played, dear, what a triumph,' he says in a shaky voice. He leans on my arms for support before tottering off to watch another match.

Peter emerges, and pats me on the back, 'Good girl, I'll be talking to you later.' He walks off, not wanting to break up the celebration.

Mrs Betty, from out of nowhere, appears and waves at me, mouthing, 'Well done.' I sometimes think she must be a ghost.

I want this feeling to last for ever.

At the end of the day it is announced over the speaker that I have won the 'Under Fourteen Girls' Match of the Day' – a pizza voucher for two. As Connie, Helen, Mum and I are piling our plates with the side salads and thousand island dressing, I cannot help thinking about the match. I have to keep reassuring myself that it is not a dream, that I really am in the last eight.

Bedtime. I can't sleep. All I can think about is winning the Nationals.

11

Rules, Rules, Rules . . .

It's July 1989, a year on from Eastbourne. I'm fifteen.

It's my last night in Delmenhorst, at the end of a South Region tour in Germany. These past two weeks have been fantastic.

I was chosen by Peter to go to Germany for two weeks with eight other South Region players, four boys, four girls. We've been playing in three-day tournaments held in Delmenhorst, Osnabrück and Wolfsburg.

I am now in the A group in the Region — Peter told me how much I had improved since making the last eight at Eastbourne (unfortunately I lost my quarter-final match, but the tournament was a breakthrough for me). For the first time I like him. And when he told me I was going to be selected for Germany, I could have kissed that curly moustache I was so happy.

We travelled in the reliable old minibus, leaving at four thirty in the morning from Bisham Abbey. In the group is a girl called Charlotte, whom I did not know very well before the tour started. She's a year older than me, she's fun, out-going and pretty — we've got on so well it feels like I've always known her.

Peter, the only way he knew how, gave us the rundown on how we should behave at the beginning of the tour. 'Lights out by ten, no girls going into the boys' rooms after ten, and remember we are here to win.

Whatever you do, don't call this a holiday.' All the correct behaviour on and off the court was spelt out to us; anyone who stepped out of line would be severely reprimanded. Charlotte and I lost our way back from the supermarket one night and were late for our evening meal. We really were lost but Peter failed to see any humour in the situation. We were late, we'd broken a rule, that's all it boiled down to.

Play starts at nine o'clock, which means a half-past seven to eight o'clock breakfast of cold meats, rubber cheese and black coffee. The tournaments have been on shale courts, which are a challenge because we are so used to playing on grass or hard. The surface is surprisingly slow compared with the British indoor fast court.

'Rallies are going to be much longer – you have got to be tough physically, expect three-hour-long matches,' Peter said during the first tournament. 'The majority of continental players are fitter, they have more stamina, they are more prepared to sustain long rallies. Look at players like Arantxa Sanchez Vicario, who runs around like a beetle, prepared to rally until her legs drop off. I want to see that from all of you. Remember, I've chosen you to be here, don't let me down. Good luck.'

I enjoy playing abroad. There isn't the endless hanging around, waiting to play your matches. Competitors can wear whatever they like, there's none of this 'predominantly whites' rule. There are also no umpires, but disputes are rare because the mark from the shale indicates whether the ball is in or out.

I have improved from practising and playing on shale, I've become much more consistent. I reached the semi-final of the last tournament, beating seeds on the way. I won a little pink hair-drier (why?) and a silver plate for being in the last four. It's a great feeling to win abroad, it builds the bricks of your confidence even more.

As a team, we've all become close, watching and supporting each other's matches. Charlotte and I have trained together, we've picked each other up after losing. Off the court, we've talked about parties we've been to, the latest films, music and people we've met through tennis.

Peter takes us all out in the evenings. He talks to us about the day and the match schedules for the following day. He has tried to get to know us and what we are like off the court. Last night he was in a foul mood with Charlotte and me because reception had charged our room a horrendous amount for use of the minibar and for watching the porn channel. 'I don't care if you're into that kind of stuff, but don't do it at my expense, have you got that?' he said, screwing up his face in anger. Trying not to laugh, Charlotte and I protested our innocence. We only had to look at the boys to know who was guilty.

It's our last night in Germany, the tournaments are over. Charlotte and I are watching television.

'Alice, change channel, you're in a daze,' Charlotte moans, grabbing the controls. 'Nothing's on. I'm not watching football or tennis. I'm really bored,' she continues. 'Let's go and annoy the boys.'

We find the boys sprawled across the floor watching the football. We jump on their bed and talk. I don't notice how late it is getting . . .

There is a knocking and the unmistakable voice of Peter behind the door. 'Have you seen the girls? They must be with you boys.' I look at my watch and panic.

Charlotte hides under the duvet, I crawl under the bed. 'They left their door slightly open. I know they are not in their room,' Peter carries on. 'Let me in, boys.'

They open the door. 'No, I haven't,' one of them stammers, looking at the other for back-up.

My heart is pounding. He will kill us. Why didn't we leave earlier? There is a long pause.

Peter says, 'Look, I know they are in here. You might as well come out, girls.'

Charlotte crawls out from under the covers; I slide out as gracefully as I can from under the bed. Charlotte and I are sitting on the floor, not sure what to do.

'Right, go to your rooms. I'll deal with the pair of you in a minute,' Peter says, making us feel as if we are pure scum of the earth, not even fit to wriggle with worms.

We go to our rooms like scolded children and collapse on to our beds, giggling nervously. We are both terrified of what our punishment will be.

When we hear Peter walking down the corridor we try to compose ourselves. 'We're really sorry, we didn't notice the time,' I try as a first excuse.

And quickly Charlotte adds, 'It was totally innocent.'

'I'm sure you weren't interested in those two clowns. I give you girls more credit. But that's not the point. You know the rules, and it's late. I'm going to have to take action,' he announces firmly.

The following day, the journey back is awkward, and what do we say when we get home? What is Peter going to do? It wasn't that bad. We deserve to be told off, but he is behaving as if we have committed a terrible crime. If he had his way we'd be on *Crimewatch UK*.

Mum and Dad are angry and disappointed in me. They

want to know how we could have been so stupid. Especially when, a week later, a letter arrives.

> *Following the rather regrettable incident on the last evening of our tour of Germany, I have to inform you that the Disciplinary Committee has met and has decided that after due consideration the following steps are to be taken:*
>
> *That each of you should be suspended from Regional training for the period of October and November, this to include all training, residential weekends, matches and tournaments.*
>
> *As I stated at the time, this Committee has not had to meet since I took over as N.C.D.O. in the South Region and I must confess that I am disappointed that we have had to take the above-mentioned steps . . .*

I am furious. I know I am in the wrong, but this punishment is totally out of proportion to what I have done. My parents are astonished that he has gone so far. It is not constructive, for a minor offence, to prevent the four of us from competing. We all write back, begging Peter to reconsider, asking him to be more lenient. However, it is all in vain. How am I going to cope with not playing tennis for two months?

Two months is so long. What am I going to do at the weekends? Suddenly I find I have too much free time on my hands. Charlotte and I visit each other and try to forget about it. We also see the funny side of it. But I miss tennis, I miss the competitions, I miss seeing Connie and I miss winning. I hate hearing who won this and who won that when I know it could have been me.

I won't let Peter do this again. I will not give him the satisfaction. I am going to be a golden girl and never step out of line. No one and nothing will stop me from playing again.

12

The Sunshine State

It's December 1989. The rivalry between Martina Navra-tilova and Chris Evert has finally come to an end. Chris Evert has retired. She won Wimbledon the year I was born and will always remain my tennis idol.

Bill is taking me plus three of his players who have had the best results in the National Championships to America for three weeks.

As the plane leaves the runway, I pinch myself to make sure it really is me going with it. Three weeks off school. I will miss Rebecca, but 'America,' I think excitedly. I hold on to my seat and turn to smile at Bill.

We arrive late and stay in the Ramada International Miami Airport Hotel. The heat at Miami airport hits you immediately – it is like stepping into a sauna.

Bill does not let us lie in on our first morning. He wants us up by eight to go running around the grounds of the hotel and afterwards we are to have a quick breakfast and then get straight out on to the practice courts.

'Bill, what are you drinking?' I ask him, watching him pour some disgusting-looking orange slush into his glass for breakfast.

'V8 juice – eight different vegetables liquidized. Delic-ious, do you want to try some?'

'Ugh, no thanks.' You always get to know people and their weird habits on holiday.

After breakfast we all head for the Miami Shores Country Club, off Sanssouci Boulevard. We have to practise for our first tournament. The heat is unbearable – ninety degrees. The sun is burning down on the courts, I feel as if I'm cooking. We do some gruelling footwork and speed exercises on the court and then begin to hit some balls. After each rally I am gasping for water – I feel dehydrated. My tennis grip turns to a wet sponge. My clothes are drenched in sweat after minutes. I dig into my tennis bag to find my tennis skirt but the pocket's empty, I forgot to put it in. Shit.

I can feel sweat trickling down my legs. Bill tells me to change. 'You must be baked, girl,' he shouts over to me.

'No, fine,' I lie. It's our first day here and I don't want to appear disorganized already.

At the end of the day my face looks scarlet and my tracksuit is clinging to me like a wetsuit. Sexy. All I want to do is jump into a tub of ice.

'My, you have caught the sun today, honey,' a lady drawls at me when I pass her in the clubhouse. 'Have you got a fever?' I pretend not to have heard. I go up to Bill, who is drinking a glass of water at the bar. 'I can't cope with this heat, it's too hot, I'll never get through a match.'

'You'll get used to it,' he says, smiling. 'But next time remember to bring your skirt,' he laughs. He knows me too well. 'What factor sun-cream are you wearing though? You need to go a lot higher.'

Our first competition, the Montanas Tournament – I am still finding the heat difficult but I play well, reaching the semi-finals. I lose to an Argentinian. The others do well, one of them reaches the Under Eighteen finals.

Their success makes me feel motivated. I want to do as well as them . . . no, I want to do better.

For the second week we stay in the Miami Marriot Hotel. It is a huge place with an indoor and outdoor swimming-pool, a gymnasium and ten tennis courts.

Breakfast is like a banquet. A long table spreads across the room, laden with scrambled, fried and poached eggs, crispy bacon, mushrooms, tomatoes, sausages, waffles, toast, Danish pastries, fruit salads, cereals and yoghurts. We walk out with bananas, yoghurts, in fact anything we can lay our hands on, poked up our sleeves.

Our second tournament is the Miami Shores Junior International Classic Tournament. There are players from Trinidad, South Africa, Zimbabwe, the USA and England. The courts are hard and fast – my favourite surface. My semi-final is a tight, three-set match. I make it to the final. I am playing a Florida-based Anglophile. I have never played her before and she is national standard. Bill has so much faith in me, he believes I can win. If I had been playing Martina Navratilova or Steffi Graf, he would have said I had a good chance. I love his optimism. I want to play well for him just as much as for me. I want to give something back.

Many people are watching the final. It is tense. She keeps screaming when she hits a bad shot. She has squinty eyes and a pinched, discontented look about her. She looks like a grumpy bulldog. She's the worst sport I have played and I don't like her at all. I have got to beat her.

'I'm playing SO badly,' she's yelling.

I win, 7–5, 7–5. Bill's flapping his arms around, frantically mouthing, 'Well done.' I am presented with a trophy and a wooden clock with a tennis player on it.

'Smile, don't look down . . . OK, another one, look at me,' Bill is saying, scurrying around the court, taking my picture like a mad Japanese man. I look up and give him a beaming smile.

That night we all go out to celebrate.

'No English player has ever won that tournament. You've got a lot to be proud of,' Bill says triumphantly, in between mouthfuls of pizza.

One more tournament to go – the Orange Bowl, held at David Park, Hollywood, a suburb of Miami. This is a huge, prestigious event. I am competing in the qualifying draw, hoping to gain a place in the main draw.

I am now staying with a local American family in a very palatial house. They have an enormous fridge filled with ice-cream of every flavour which I frequently find myself eating. The boys do not fare nearly as well and moan at Bill every time I am dropped off at the gates, passing the security guards.

My qualifying match is disappointing. I lose to a Venezuelan girl 6–4, 6–4. I played badly. I need to be more professional and not be intimidated by the big events. I still have so much to learn.

We spend the last few days soaking up the sun on the beach, training, shopping. We watch Jennifer Capriati playing in a tournament. I'd love to come here again, play more tournaments, defend my title at Miami Shores and qualify for the Orange Bowl. I'd love to come to America again.

'There's no reason why you shouldn't come back, Alice,' Bill says. 'America won't go away. It's up to you and how much you want it.'

13

The Red Carnation

It's April. I'm sixteen. I have reached the semi-finals of the Under Sixteen, Prudential Junior Hard Court Championships of Great Britain 1990, held by the LTA on the hard courts, red shale, of West Hants Lawn Tennis Club, Bournemouth.

I'm ranked number one in the South Region Under Sixteen and Eighteen. If I win today, I will be seeded in the top eight in the country. I have so much to play for.

Dad watched me beat the number seven seed yesterday. It was one of the first times he came to support me. He has never been into the tennis scene but I know he enjoyed it. It opened his eyes to how high the standard was, we don't just plop it over the net delicately, scared of breaking our nails.

Dad was praying desperately for me to win yesterday. I looked up and could see his hands clenched together, his head down.

'Dad, were you praying for me?! Did you watch any of my match? Your head was always down!' I asked him after the match. He just smiled, not saying anything. I could see a few extra grey hairs on his head too – I don't think Dad likes to watch because he gets too uptight. 'Well, it must have worked, keep on praying.' Dad's been my lucky charm.

★

'Bill, hi,' I say, opening the front door.

'How are you feeling, nervous?'

'Very.'

'You don't need to be. I think you can win.' He hands me an envelope. Inside is a red carnation. 'It's for luck. Meet in half an hour for some practice before the big match, OK?'

After Bill has gone, I sit down on the stairs and read his letter.

> *Dear Alice*
>
> *Congratulations! What an achievement. So many people dream about just getting to the Nationals and now you have reached the last four. You are, without question, one of the best young lady players in Britain, a fact which everyone must recognize. You've succeeded through effort, skill, courage and good sense and you are such a credit to the game and Hampshire tennis in particular.*
>
> *You have nothing more to prove. It is obvious you are an outstanding competitor and player and now you can test yourself and see just how far you can go. Give it everything you have and from now on allow your natural talents to move you forward into exciting territory.*
>
> *You have already surprised many people in tennis; now play like you've never played before and surprise even yourself.*
>
> *You can do it; have fun and belt the ball only you know how.*
>
> *Love and luck Bill.*

After reading his letter, it finally sinks in that all the effort, the training, the travelling has been worth it. I am in a wonderful, exciting position and have everything to go for.

I am playing a girl from South Wales today, also unseeded. This tournament has knocked out virtually all the seeds. We, the players, have been singing in Freddie Mercury style, 'Another seed bites the dust.'

I know I can win. She is expected to win on paper but I am not nearly so much in awe of other players any more – I feel I am up with the 'big girls', I have as good a chance as any of them to do well. So much depends on who plays well on the day. Everything is familiar now – the format, the umpiring, the faces. I still feel nervous but once I'm on the court, into the match, I know I'll be fine. I enjoy it, although Mum always says I look miserable on court, as if I'm being punished. It's only because I'm concentrating so hard. We all look like that.

If I win, my picture will be in newspapers and I will be in the final, where we are presented with flowers before the match like at Wimbledon. I want to win so much because nobody expects me to, I am the underdog.

Bill winks at me, saying, 'Good luck, we're all rooting for you,' as I walk on to the court. The red carnation is with me, tucked into the pocket of my racket bag.

Peter is watching, along with many other spectators. Connie and Charlotte, Dad, Bill, Mum, who had a large vodka and tonic beforehand, the County Organizer with her fiery red hair sticking out and her eyes sparkling – she told me earlier how 'simply marvellous' it would be for Hampshire if I won.

The girl I am playing has long blonde hair, shiny white teeth and is wearing light pink lipstick. She also grunts every time she hits the ball. It doesn't seem to go with her pretty image. She is a 'hacker', a 'moonballer' – some-one who, annoyingly, gets everything back.

We have an official umpire who tosses a coin to see who has the choice of serving or receiving.

The match is hard, the rallies long. We are both tense. I do not relax at all in the first set, losing it easily. I can see anxious faces, Dad can't watch any more. Sometimes I hate people, especially Mum, watching. I know she thinks I'm playing badly. I am trying, it's just that nothing is going my way.

I play much better in the second set. I've loosened up. I'm winning four games to love.

Four games all. What has happened? The match is slipping through my fingers. She is just getting everything back. Five four to her.

'Come on,' Bill is mouthing to me at changeover. I can't lose, this girl is no better than me. It should be one set all.

The last game is fought out, both of us playing well, but she wins. She deserved to win, she played better on the day. I feel bitterly disappointed. I wanted to win, maybe too much.

'Bad luck, love. It was a good match, nothing to be ashamed of,' says Mum, trying to offer some words of comfort although I can see she is also deeply disappointed. Mum is just as competitive as me. 'Never mind,' she continues, knowing the car journey home is going to be awful. She tells me it's like sitting next to a thundercloud when I've lost.

'It's only a game,' says Dad, not knowing how to comfort, and then wishes he'd just kept quiet when he sees my horrified expression. I walk past all of them, saying nothing.

How can he say, 'It's only a game?' It is the end of the world. They don't know anything. I don't feel like talking to anyone, not to Bill, not to Mum or Dad. I want to be on my own.

14

The Wimbledon Championships

April 1990: a week after Bournemouth. I am playing the Under Eighteen Nationals at Wimbledon. Most of the players from Bournemouth are here, along with the older girls. We are not playing our matches on the sacred grass courts, we play on the shale courts tucked away in the background of the club.

It's day three of the tournament. I won my first match. One thing this tournament has in common with THE Wimbledon Championships is the rain. It has rained for three consecutive days and everybody is bored to tears with the endless hanging around. The Tournament Organizers are pulling their hair out in frustration.

Connie and I and a few other friends are playing cards in the clubhouse, surrounded in glory by pictures of the most famous players – Connors, McEnroe, Borg, Chris Evert, Steffi, Martina, Agassi, Becker. It's awe-inspiring and one of them may even have been sitting in this exact spot.

Despite the solid rain, it's been worth it. This is one of the most important tournaments for national players to enter. The winners receive a lot of prestige and coverage. It is a step nearer to playing at THE Wimbledon. Soaking up the atmosphere, visiting the holy Centre Court, I long to come back, but come back as *THE* Alice. I long to come back for the real thing . . .

I walk through the entrance gates of the All England Club. Cameras are flashing, people are longing to catch a glimpse of me. They rush home that evening, saying, 'I saw her, I saw Alice Peterson!' Walking on to Centre Court, I allow the thunderous roar of clapping to envelop me. Thousands of people have paid to watch me. The ball-boy nervously hands me my green and purple towel along with a glass of Robinson's lemon barley water. After the match, I stride off court triumphant, crowds of screaming fans waving their pens and programmes at me. I feature on the Wimbledon Highlights at the end of the day, serving in slow motion to Jean-Michel Jarre's 'Oxygen', and the following morning I am on the front page of every newspaper, the most flattering picture of course, with the headline, '*Alice in Winnerland*'. I go on to win the finals and clamber up the stalls to my gorgeously handsome and supportive husband, who gives me a huge kiss. I clamber back down to be presented with my plate and a big fat cheque. I curtsey in front of the Duchess of Kent, who shakes me warmly by the hand, saying, 'I'm so thrilled you won.' After an invigorating shower in the famous locker-room I am chauffeur-driven back in a limousine to my luxury apartment in Chelsea, where my plate joins all the other trophies in my glass cabinet. In the evening there is a party for the players. I look positively radiant, my dress sparkling. In between being fed strawberries and cream by my wonderful husband, I am swept off the dance floor by the men's champion, Agassi every time . . .

*

Back to reality. Bump.

I lost my second round to Shirli-Ann Siddall, who is, I think, one of the most talented players in our age group. I wouldn't be surprised if she wins the tournament and comes back here for real.

Well, I can carry on dreaming. Maybe next time . . .

15

College Life

It's September 1990. I'm now at a sixth-form college, Peter Symonds, reading English, Spanish and French.

I love the freedom. I enjoy going out with boys, going to college parties and balls. I'm learning photography, going to drama classes, doing things I've never done before.

And I have fallen in love. His name's Seb. We met in our French class. He sat next to me and said, 'You're the tennis player, aren't you?' That was all he had to say. I knew instantly. He's a gorgeous distraction – tall, broad, blond hair, innocent blue eyes.

Through Seb I met a girl called Sophie. I used to tease him at first, saying he must fancy her because she's so pretty. The three of us begin to go out regularly with groups of friends to smoky pubs and karaokes. We play tennis together. We become soulmates. In the summer, we lie out on the college lawn talking about what we want to do when we're older and the people we've met through our courses. Sophie's reading psychology and loves analysing people. When she's serious, she plays with her long, dark brown, almost black, hair and bites her lower lip, wrinkling her nose like a rabbit. She is frighteningly perceptive – I feel she understands me already.

I go on holiday with Sophie and Seb and a few others to France at the beginning of the summer. I plan to combine the holiday with a few tennis tournaments in France, as I need to keep up the practice for the nationals in August.

As the end of our holiday draws near, I find that in many ways I do not want to leave. I love eating lots of French bread and chocolate, the late-night swims in the sea, staying up late and talking around the fire, and being close to Seb.

For the first time I'm thinking about someone more than tennis.

16

America!

September 1991: Steffi Graf and Michael Stich won Wimbledon this year. Why are the Germans so good at tennis? We need a British champion.

I'm waiting for a lady to call round and tell me about a tennis scholarship in America. She's an agent who works for the Prospects of America scheme. She rang last week, wanting to know whether I had ever considered the idea of a tennis scholarship in the USA.

America! I could travel, be away from home, be independent. I could meet new people, perhaps even meet the man of my dreams. I'd be able to keep up my tennis as well as study for a degree. Charlotte's in America now and tells me the coaching is wonderful – her coach is encouraging and laid back, but pushes her hard. And she's fallen in love. I want to be there too.

We hear a car coming up the drive. 'It's bound to be someone to see you, isn't it?' Tom says snidely and starts stomping up the stairs.

'What is it with him? He ought to be happy for me, I would be for him . . .' I start to say, but Mum stops me. 'Just leave it, Alice, you know what he's like,' she says sharply. 'He'll calm down.' As Tom reaches his bedroom the door slams and loud music is turned on.

Rain is pelting down against the door. Mum lets a

dark-haired woman in. She wipes her feet on the doormat and shakes her umbrella out.

'Oh, you poor thing, you're soaked,' Mum says. 'Come on inside, let me take your coat.'

I can hear their voices and start to feel anxious about the interview.

'One good reason to go to America is to get away from the weather here,' she laughs, sitting down.

'I know, it's dreadful,' I agree. Mum comes in to join us with our coffees.

'OK, Alice, this is how I can help you. If you decide to go to America, going through me makes things easier. I will do a profile on you. Coaches like to see a photograph accompanied by a short biography including details of your education. With the tennis, they will want to know your strengths and weaknesses, your rankings. Once we have done that it will get passed around. We just wait and see what response we get. It's as easy as that.'

'And you charge a fee,' Mum reminds her. I think she trusts the agent but she has to bring up the practical side of things, a side I tend to forget.

'In the region of three hundred pounds. It may seem a lot, but in the past I have had terrific results. All the young sports people I have dealt with have been extremely happy with the whole procedure. If you go through us, you are more likely to get to the college of your choice because of our contacts. Do you think this interests you, Alice?'

'Yes, definitely,' I reply impulsively.

'It would be a wonderful opportunity. I'm nervous about her going away, though, she may never come back,' Mum says.

She chuckles. 'All parents say that, but it is one of the best ways to combine academic study with competitive, tournament tennis. Well, we can get started right away.' She pulls out some forms from her leather case. Her gold chunky bracelet slides up and down her wrist. It matches her necklace and gold belt.

'What's your date of birth?' she asks. Mum slips out of the room, I imagine she'll go upstairs to see Tom.

'25.1.74.'

We go through all the basic questions about my education up to date. The tennis comes last.

'What standard are you?'

'National.'

'Excellent. Ranking in County?'

'Number one.'

'Regional?'

'Number one.'

'National?'

'I was seeded eight in the last tournament at Eastbourne.'

She's scribbling it down. 'Your rankings are great. Once all this information gets processed, I'd expect coaches either to ring you at home or send you a letter. Now, do you know anything about the SAT exam?'

'A little.' I know nothing about it but I don't want to appear stupid.

'SAT stands for Scholastic Assessment Test. You have to sit the SAT 1 test, a three hour paper, primarily multiple choice.' She hands me some past papers. 'It's quite different from exams here. It's just Maths and English, designed to assess basic verbal and mathematical reasoning.' She sounds like a textbook. 'You will have to sit the exam in December or January. Don't worry, you have plenty of time to prepare. Here's some information about the colleges for you to read. Oh, one last thing. Do you have a photograph? One of you in action on the court would be the best.'

I run upstairs to my bedroom, tripping up on the way, and flip through my album. Tom comes in and says sorry. 'I like that one,' he suggests, his clumsy fingers pointing to a picture of me playing tennis when I was in Spain. 'I was talking to Mum,' Tom says. 'I am glad you've got this chance. You're my sister. I want you to be happy.'

'It's all right,' I say quickly, too excited to say anything more. I slide the photo out and rush back down the stairs.

'Perfect,' she gushes, taking the photograph. 'Your profile will be very good, I feel very confident that we can find you an excellent college.'

We show her to the door. When she's out of sight, I turn round to hug Mum. 'This is fantastic. I can't believe I might go to America. I know it's what I want.'

I am sitting by the phone waiting for a call.

'It's far too early yet,' Mum says. The phone rings.

'Hi, can I speak with a Miss Alice Peterson?'

'Oh hi, this is Alice,' I reply, my voice rising unnaturally. Keep calm and cool, I tell myself, flicking the elastic band on my wrist.

'Well, hi there, Alice. It's Stuart Martin, I'm the tennis coach at Ohio. I'm sure you know why I'm calling. I've seen your profile. We sure liked it over here. We think you'd be an asset to our team. Have you had any other offers yet?'

'No, this is my first call.' Shit, why did I say that? Make them believe the offers are flooding in.

'I'm real glad. We are one of the best colleges in America. You need look no further.'

I cringe in my seat, although I'm enjoying the conversation.

He goes on to describe the facilities, the countryside, the tennis tournaments they play in. 'Think about us, Alice, we'll be in touch.' We hang up.

The phone rings again.

'Hi, it's Coach Peterson calling from Louisiana. Looks like we have something in common already! Alice, I'd love to talk to you about our college . . .'

I just have time to make myself a sandwich before the phone rings again. Mayonnaise is dribbling down my cheek, my hands are so greasy I drop the receiver.

'Calling from Virginia, Alice, are you there, Alice?' I put the receiver to my ear quickly again.

That week many offers come in, each more pushy than the last.

'Our area is streaks ahead of anywhere else. You'd be crazy to miss a golden opportunity like this . . .' advises Al from Denver.

'You must play a great game of tennis, hit that ball real hard. I liked your profile. I sure hope you might consider coming to us in the fall . . .' says Walt Wiseman, calling from Tennessee.

'Our team is the best in the States. We have the finest reputation,' says another.

'Our facilities are state of the art.'

'We are the best, we want you. Choose us, Alice.'

My head is expanding by the second to the size of an enormous beach-ball. They want me. I love it.

I like the coach at Louisiana, Coach Peterson. She

talked about her college and the way she coached without being pushy. Louisiana is definitely in the lead.

My agent calls, telling me my SAT exam is scheduled for 25 January.

'That's my birthday,' I realize. 'That's really annoying. I can't change it, can I?'

'Alice, really, this is your SAT exam. I'd also like you to make a video. Play and talk – let them get an idea of your personality. We'll send it to Louisiana first.'

Bill is at the club, setting the video machine up.

'I'm nervous,' I say, doing a few warm-up exercises. 'OK, I'm ready, Bill.'

'Brush your hair. You look as if you've rolled out of the bushes. Come on, Alice, we've got to impress.'

'OK, OK!' I say, clipping my hair back again. I'm wearing my black Donnay tracksuit with its rainbow logo and I have a few new blonde highlights in my hair. I think I look really smart actually.

Take One:

'Hi there, we're going to watch Alice Peterson play today. A short interview will also give you an idea of what she's like as a person.' Bill turns towards me, 'Alice, what sort of standard have you achieved in tennis?'

I tell him I qualified to play in the Under Eighteen Dewhurst Cup Masters at Queen's Club with the top fourteen players in the country.

'To qualify you must have had some terrific results against some of the top juniors. You beat Shirli-Ann Siddall at Wimbledon, didn't you? What a great result.'

I stare at him. He knows I didn't beat her. What's he doing? Bill realizes he's gone wrong. 'Lie,' he's mouthing.

'I didn't beat her, this is dreadful, cut it. Bill, cut.'

Bill fumbles around, eventually pressing the stop button.

Take Two:

'Where do you see yourself going in the next two, three years?' Bill asks.

'I will go to America. I think I could really go for it out there. I feel I would have more of a chance of making it to the top, to Wimbledon.'

'Have you been to America before?'

I stare at him again. 'Yes, with you.' Dipstick.

'Excellent, excellent. And you're not a one-dimensional character, you want to keep up your study?'

'Yes, I hope to read psychology and keep up my languages. I enjoy the arts.' I feel as if I'm on Miss World. I ought to be saying, 'I love to travel and I love animals,' with my Miss Winchester ribbon around me, in my swim-suit and with a crown on my head.

Time to play. I walk to the other side of the court. First shot in the net.

'Edit that out please,' I say, smiling.

It's 25 January, my eighteenth birthday. Dad drops me off in London to sit my SAT exam. I walk along the crowded corridor – people are pushed up against the wall like sardines. We are organized into groups and taken to the room where we sit the three-hour exam. The exam is divided into six half-hour sections. The Maths sections include fractions, decimals, ratios, powers and roots, geometry, equations. The English sections include sentence-correcting, comprehension, selecting words which mean the same as the one underlined, ringing antonyms. It sounds simple but you have to work quickly and it is easy to make mistakes. The highest score is 1,600. I need to get 1,000 plus to get into Louisiana. If I don't get the points, I don't get in. I have to put everything into this exam. I cannot imagine not going to America now. I must pass.

After the exam I head straight for the tube station – I'm meeting Helen at Covent Garden. My right hand is hurting, my head feels like cotton wool. Helen, where are you? Thank goodness she's tall, I think, immediately spotting her among the crowds outside the station.

'I'll miss your funny face when you go to America,' Helen says, drinking a glass of wine in a bar. My right hand is still aching. It must be from all the writing. 'How did it go?' she asks.

'I can't tell, their vocab is weird. Anyway, it's over. Will you miss me?'

'You know I will. Keep in touch all the time. You never know, you might meet a handsome American and stay out there for the rest of your life.'

'Hope so,' I say dreamily.

'Mum's scared you'll never come back. I will miss you, you're my best friend . . . it will be very strange without you.' She takes another sip of wine. 'Al, you've been rubbing your hand the whole time.'

'Am I?' I hadn't noticed. 'Oh, it just feels a bit funny.' I stop rubbing it.

'Must be sore after all that scribbling,' Helen decides.

'How's the new job going, by the way?' Helen is working for a design company in London. She is a trained graphic designer.

'Oh, it's all right. I want a pay rise though! Anyway I'm bored of talking to you, let's go shopping.' She gets up, bill in her hand, and strides confidently to the bar in her leather jacket, jeans and heeled boots. My sister is too trendy.

We leave the bar and link arms, walking towards the market.

We go to a hat stall and try on practically every hat. Helen buys a black Russian hat and picks out a dark green floppy velvet one for me.

'I've got to get you that,' she insists, standing back.

We drive back to Winchester, the back seat cluttered with shopping bags. My right hand is still aching. I quickly forget about it and start thinking about my party at home that evening. I feel happy because my SAT exam is over. Tonight I want to enjoy myself.

Seb, Sophie and her boyfriend stay the night after my party. We all crash out in my room. Sophie is snoring, keeping everyone awake.

Seb and I can't sleep. 'I got you this.' Seb hands me a little bag. Inside is a silver puzzle ring. 'Do you like it? I haven't had much experience of buying girls presents.'

'I love it . . . I love you,' I whisper.

'I'll miss you. Are you really going to America?'

'If I get the right results, yes.' I lie back, holding his hand. Sophie snores again.

'Yes, I am going to America.'

Life is perfect.

17

'It hurts, Mum'

It's February 1992. Jim Courier beats Stefan Edberg in the Australian Open. Monica Seles wins the women's title.

'Mum, my thumb hurts.'

She looks at it.

'I can't grip my racket properly.' I clench my hand into a fist and open it out again. The feeling is hard to describe; it isn't painful, it just feels weak. I begin to rub it.

Mum says, 'It's a little bruised, but it's not swollen. What do you think it could be?'

Suddenly I remember yesterday, Seb pushing me up the wall and through my bedroom window because we were locked out of the house. I scraped my hand badly. That must be it. I smile, remembering how we got the giggles when I was standing on his shoulders and he nearly dropped me. 'I don't know. I'll go to the club, knock a few balls around, see if I can play.'

'OK, but if it hurts you should pull out of the match.'

'Yes, Mum,' I say in a tone which implies, 'Stop nagging. I wish I hadn't told you.'

We arrive at the club. I see my doubles partner looking eager to play. She hasn't seen me yet, so I walk quickly round to the back of the clubhouse to hit a ball against the wall.

I take the racket out of my bag. I still cannot hold it properly, it's going to be impossible to play. I lean against the wall. I stare at my hand, prod it around. I'll really let her down, I think, we should win the final, this is ridiculous. The prize money is good too.

As I walk back to the clubhouse, I hear our names being called out on the loudspeaker. I head straight towards my partner and tell her there is something wrong with my hand. She is kind, concerned – she used to be a nurse and suggests I go down to Casualty to have it checked out. This seems over the top. I mean, it's not really an emergency, is it? But Mum agrees.

At the Casualty Department the waiting-room is hectic with phones ringing, people drifting in and out, ambulances pulling up outside. I feel disappointed and stupid. I've never had to pull out of a match before, never.

There are children crying, sullen faces, old and young, blood and bandages. There is a sense of urgency, panic; I feel a fraud with my little thumb, embarrassed to make a fuss. 'This is such a hassle. Why did we bother? We'll have to wait ages,' I moan. I hate doctors. One of the few times I saw my GP, complaining about bad, hammering headaches, he looked at me suspiciously and said, 'And when do the headaches come on? When it is time to do the washing up?' 'Can't we go home? It feels better now.'

Mum ignores me.

I am called. No escape now. I sit down in the cubicle, the curtain is drawn around us for privacy.

The doctor comes in. 'Now, what can I do for you?'

'Oh, it's just my thumb, I can't grip anything,' I reveal casually.

'Let me have a look. Perhaps you've just strained it.'

'Yes, that's what I thought. I scraped it yesterday. I'm sure it's nothing serious.'

He straps it up in a tight bandage which I want to rip off, it feels uncomfortable. 'I don't think it's anything to worry about but keep an eye on it. Come back if the pain persists. I'll give you a few mild painkillers in the meantime.'

We go home. I cheer up, slouched on the sofa watching the *Brookside* omnibus and *Blind Date*.

The next day my thumb is fine, the pain in my hand has vanished. I go up to the tennis club and play as if nothing had happened.

Two weeks later, 7 a.m. I hurry into my parents' room. Dad and Mum are awake, drinking their early morning tea.

'What on earth's the matter?' Mum asks. 'Alice, darling, what's wrong? Why are you up so early?'

'It's my wrist. I can't move it,' I say, tears streaming down my face. The pain is sharp, biting.

Mum looks anxious but remains calm. 'Ssh, calm down,' she says gently. 'Go and get dressed and we'll go to Casualty again.'

I try to put my clothes on without moving my wrist. The slightest movement hurts.

Back at Casualty I'm seen quite quickly. I tell the doctor I play tennis, could it be anything related to that? He says he's not worried, it's probably a strain injury but I ought to be seen by a hand and wrist specialist at the hospital and have an X-ray to be on the safe side. He calls the specialist for an appointment. 'It shouldn't be long. We'll send an appointment card to you.'

The next day my wrist doesn't hurt at all, I've been making a fuss about nothing. I'm sure everybody gets aches and pains now and then, even me.

Coach Peterson is on the line again. 'Hi, how are you?' she asks.

'Great,' I reply.

'Thank you very much for making the video. I've discussed you with a few of the other coaches and I would love to offer you a place, Alice, provided you get the required SAT results. I would love to have you on our team.'

I put the phone down and ring Helen immediately.

'That's great! You clever thing, bet Mum and Dad are pleased.'

'They are, we all are!'

'Oh, by the way, is your hand OK now?'

'Yes, yes it's fine. It was just a strain injury, something like that.'

'Weird . . . well, at least it's better.'

I ring Sophie, I ring Seb. I want to ring the whole world. Seb cycles over to play tennis with me. In the evening we celebrate, stealing a bottle of Dad's champagne.

It is now March. I am helping Bill coach a group of adults at the club.

'Alice, can you do a demo serve?' Bill asks.

I hit a couple of serves. My shoulder is hurting. It does not like the overarm action.

'Alice? Are you all right? I saw you wincing a few times when you hit your serve.'

'I think I've pulled a muscle. But I can't remember straining it. I've been having a few problems recently . . . Oh, I'm sure it's nothing.'

Bill looks at my shoulder. 'You look tired. You need to go home, have a hot bath, supper and bed.'

'Yes, my English coursework will just have to wait.' I go home, eagerly anticipating a hot bubble bath.

The next day my shoulder pain has disappeared completely.

At college, a week later, Seb, Sophie, a friend and I are playing mixed doubles. I can't do an overarm at all now; I can't lift my shoulders, which feel like heavy bricks. I do a pathetic underarm which dribbles over the net. This is the great tennis player who played the Nationals at Wimbledon. What is going on? I watch another serve plop off the racket. Seb must think I'm so bad. Sophie asks me if I'm OK. I laugh it off but this is really annoying me. Can I really say it's nothing?

I go back to Seb's house for supper and afterwards we lie on his bed, I take my top off and he rubs some Deep Heat into my shoulders. No romantic aromatherapy oils for me. It stinks. 'I'm worried about you.' Seb kisses me. 'You haven't been yourself. You are all right aren't you? Has the Deep Heat helped?'

'Yes, but carry on. I love massage and it's really working,' I lie. We get through practically the whole tube.

Mum makes an appointment for me to go and see the GP again.

'With all the symptoms you describe it could be galloping arthritis,' he says, pricking me with the sharp needle and drawing out more dark blood.

'No way,' I dismiss. 'Only old people get that.'

A day later my GP phones with the results, which are negative. Phew. The phone rings again immediately. It's my American agent with the SAT results.

'Alice, you did OK, you got enough points to go to

Louisiana, congratulations. All your hard work has paid off.'

Everything is wonderful. I'm sure I've just been stressed about my results for America, and my A levels which are in a couple of months. But I don't need to worry about anything now. Louisiana will accept me! Everything is piecing together.

Coach Peterson is on the line. 'I've just had the results. I'm so pleased you'll be joining us. A contract will be drawn up. Well done. Keep up with the match play over the summer, all I want you to do now is maintain your level of fitness.'

It's approaching Easter. The aches and pains have been darting around my body, but they are mainly in my hands and wrists. Then they disappear, lulling me into a false sense of security, making me think I've been imagining it all.

I crawl across the landing, dragging myself to the loo. My body feels as if it's wading through thick boggy mud. I have no energy.

'Alice, what are you doing?' Mum gasps, looking down at me. 'Right, that's it, you've got to be seen now.'

I am scared. What's wrong with my body? Why does it feel like this? Why do I feel so tired?

Mum phones the hospital, saying I have to be seen straight away – we aren't prepared to wait any longer, we'll go private if we have to. 'She must have another blood test before the appointment too. I can't believe nothing is wrong, it isn't normal,' she stresses. She manages to get an appointment.

I am seeing the specialist at the hand and wrist clinic

today and nothing hurts. Typical. But there must be something wrong. I know I am not a fraud.

We are sitting in the specialist's waiting-room. I am called in and see a young doctor, slumped in his chair. He looks half asleep. I think he must have a huge hangover. He examines my wrist first. 'Does this hurt?' he asks.

'No.'

'This?' He yanks it the other way and yawns.

'No.'

'Well, there doesn't seem to be much wrong,' he concludes, leaning back into his chair.

'It's not just my wrist. I haven't been feeling well. And the pains dart around.'

'Um,' he mutters, not convinced.

This is getting nowhere. 'Have you had the results of my last blood test?' I ask.

He picks up the phone. 'Right, yes, I'll give pathology a call. Miss A. Peterson, her results please. Thank you.'

He scribbles down the results and then puts the phone down slowly.

'Well?'

'The tests show you have . . .' He pauses.

'What?'

'Rheumatoid arthritis.'

18

What is Rheumatoid Arthritis?

Thank goodness, I've got rheumatoid arthritis. I'm not a fraud. I can see the rheumatologist tomorrow, treat it and make it better. I can get on with life again. At least I know what it is.

Mum and I drive back in silence.

I am walking down the airy, rather depressing long corridors. A smell of stale cabbage drifts from the kitchens. Mum and I pass porters pushing frail-looking people in wheelchairs, doctors in white coats, nurses and visitors. Mum is fighting back the tears. I have a spring to my step, I want to be seen quickly. I laugh and tell Mum to keep up with me.

We walk down another set of corridors, the walls decorated with colourful paintings of ducks and ponds and other farm animals. In the lift we press A for the Rheumatology Department.

We are in the waiting-room, where everyone else is considerably older than me. A lady wearing a fur hat is parked next to me in a wheelchair. She presents her appointment card and there's a look of horror on her face when the nurse says she has to be weighed.

A small lady with white curly hair sits hunched in her wheelchair opposite me. She lifts her head, stares at me blankly and then looks down again. For the first time I feel uneasy.

A nurse gives me a plastic pot and asks for a urine sample. Going for a pee kills five minutes.

Another nurse hands me a form to fill in and I skim over some of the questions:

- *Are you able to dress yourself, including tying shoelaces and doing buttons?*
- *Open a new carton of milk (or soap powder)?*
- *Lift a full cup or glass to your mouth?*
- *Stand up from an armless straight chair?*
- *Run errands and shop?*

Beside each question I have the choice of ticking, 'Without ANY difficulty,' 'With SOME difficulty,' 'With MUCH difficulty,' or 'Unable to do.'

'Mum, these questions are ridiculous. Of course I can lift a cup to my mouth!' I say incredulously, ticking, 'Without ANY difficulty' for each one.

'I suppose for some people it must be difficult otherwise they wouldn't ask those questions,' Mum says softly.

I'm staring at the sugar pink walls. The round clock, with large white and black numbers, says three o'clock. I look beyond the waiting area to the ward, where the pace of activity is frantic, with phones ringing constantly and nurses rushed off their feet.

Eventually at 3.40 p.m. I am called. Dr Buckley shakes our hands, beckoning my mother and me to sit down. We whisk through all the polite questions – how old am I, where am I at college? He's Canadian. He asks me about my tennis and the scholarship to America. 'I play tennis but my wife tells me I'm too slow around the court. Need to get rid of this,' he laughs, poking his stomach. He then confirms that my blood tests show the rheumatoid. 'Do you know anything about it?' he asks, looking at both Mum and me.

'No, not much,' I reply.

'Rheumatoid arthritis is a common inflammatory disease of the joints which can affect anyone of any age, but it most often begins in young women aged twenty to forty.'

'I thought it was grannies who got arthritis,' I say.

'There are hundreds of different types of arthritis, affecting people of all different ages – young children can have arthritis, babies can be born with arthritis.'

'So which one is rheumatoid arthritis then?' I ask curiously.

'It's thought to be an auto-immune disease – the body is attacking its own immune system. Antibodies and immune cells which should defend against infection do the opposite, they damage the body's own joint tissue.' He starts drawing a diagram. 'The normal joint has a smooth layer of cartilage overlying the bone end.' He points to it. 'This makes movement easy. And surrounding the joint is a layer of tissue called the synovium; this secretes a thickish fluid which lubricates the cartilage . . .'

He's scribbling down some picture. He is attractive. He's friendly. He reminds me of Jimmy Connors. I like him. At least my doctor is good-looking.

'All of this is surrounded by a capsule and ligaments which keep the joint healthy and stable,' he continues, drawing more lines.

What is he going on about now? Actually he reminds me more of Alec Baldwin. What a shame he's married.

'Whereas normal joints move freely, with rheumatoid arthritis the synovial tissue lining joints and tendons becomes chronically inflamed. This causes heat, swelling and pain . . .'

Blah blah blah. Just give me the medicine, I want to say. No more medical jargon. I want a pill or something.

'But why,' Mum stresses, wrinkles creasing her forehead, 'should a young, healthy eighteen-year-old get a condition like this? It's so out of the blue.'

'Rheumatoid arthritis can start for no obvious reason. Sometimes it is triggered off by an infection, a virus, but the exact cause is still not known.'

'And the treatment?' Mum asks.

'It can be controlled with a variety of pills – you have to shop around to see which cocktail suits you best. In many cases it will burn out, go away completely, hopefully before it has caused too much damage to the bones and joints.' He puts a hand through his hair.

'Well, now I know what it is I can treat it, can't I? As long as it clears up so I can go to America that's fine,' I say.

'Look, Alice,' he says softly, 'there are no guarantees.'

'What do you mean? The pills will help, won't they?'

'They may control it.'

'I have to go to America this autumn. That gives me all summer to rest and get better. You can get me better by then . . . can't you?' I persevere.

'Let's put you on naproxen, an anti-inflammatory. It should decrease swelling and pain. Perhaps,' his tone tentative, 'you should think about deferring for a year. Then we can . . .'

'No!' I interrupt. This idea is inconceivable. 'It will burn out, won't it?' I look to Mum for reassurance. Dr Buckley is silent. 'Can you get me better at all?' I gasp.

'Alice, I'm afraid there is no cure,' he says, hardly able to look me in the eyes.

Bombshell.

'We are going to hit it hard on the head, age is on your side. Don't think the worst yet . . .'

I can't listen properly. I feel numb. This can't be happening.

Dr Buckley reaches into his drawer and pulls out a form. He stamps his name on the front of each piece of paper like a librarian. 'I want X-rays of all your joints, and you must see an occupational therapist, she'll make you some splints. Are you OK?' he asks, looking into our white faces. I nod.

Dr Buckley gets up. Mum and I follow him like shadows. He looks at me. 'Take this,' he says, shoving a leaflet on rheumatoid arthritis into my hand.

I shake myself up, pull myself together. 'Thank you,' I reply. On the front page is a young woman with a beaming smile. Underneath she writes, 'Dear Reader, it can be devastating to be told you have rheumatoid arthritis, especially if you are in the prime of your life . . .' She looks so healthy and radiant, as if she's just been on a Caribbean holiday. We walk out of his office.

Mum and I go straight to the X-ray Department. The waiting-room is packed. Workers in maroon outfits with white belts keep coming in and out of the X-ray rooms lethargically calling out names. A boy on crutches sits next to me, his leg in plaster from his ankle to the top of his thigh. A porter pushes an old man lying on his bed into the waiting area. He is as white as the blankets covering him. There are lots of children, a few playing with the toys at the end of the room, one wailing on his mother's lap with a bandage around his wrist. Everything feels surreal, as if it isn't me in this situation.

'She won't believe it,' I say, staring into space. 'Coach Peterson won't believe it if I have to defer. It will burn out, won't it, Mum?' I ask desperately.

Before Mum has time to answer, my name is called out and I am handed a white towelling robe. 'Slip this on in one of the cubicles and then come on through,' she says, pointing to the orange door.

I walk past the waiting-room in my furry white robe and enter the X-ray room. I lie on the hard bed. Equipment hangs above me.

'So, Miss Peterson, what have we here. Um, rheumatoid arthritis.' He looks at me. 'You're a bit young, aren't you, to have something like that?' he asks in a tone which doesn't expect a reply. 'OK, place your hands on the film, and hold . . .'

I look at my right hand. It has a few bits of hard skin on the palms from playing tennis. The fingers are long and my nails are chipped, but it's strong. It is impossible to imagine that anything malign is taking place inside it – it still looks the same to me. There's nothing the matter with me.

'Hold . . . click. Hold . . . click . . .'

I pull up the robe to expose my knees. I feel bare, declothed, invaded. There's nothing wrong with my knees. Stop poking them, prodding them. Stop TOUCHING me.

Hands, feet, neck, knees and hips are all X-rayed in turn. My body is examined like a piece of machinery, bit by bit. I long to go home.

Next, Mum and I follow the signs to the Occupational Therapy Department like tourists in a foreign country.

The occupational therapy room is open-plan, the walls covered with complicated anatomy posters. Girls dressed in green trouser-suits are scuttling in and out.

We sit down at a table. I can see a pale, flesh-coloured splint with Velcro fasteners on the next table. It is ugly. The therapist notices me eyeing it with fear. 'Yes, that's what yours will look like,' she says apprehensively. She begins to draw around my hands to get the measurements right. I cannot believe I will wear a thing like that.

'Splints are used for several different reasons. You need to protect and support the joints. If joints become inflamed it is important to rest them, keep them still until the inflammation goes down, and the splints also help to keep the joints in line.' She reaches for my right hand. 'We want the fingers to remain as straight as possible, and hand splints will help prevent deformity. I am going to make you a resting splint for the night, OK, but you can wear it during the day too.'

I don't want to wear it at all.

The therapist reads my thoughts. 'I know these splints are not fashionable, far from it. You're young, they are the last things you want to wear. My younger sister has arthritis and she feels the same. I'm really sorry, it must be such a shock, the last thing you were expecting,' she says sympathetically. Her eyes look enormous, magnified through her pink-rimmed round glasses. 'Wear the splints when you are on your own during the day and at night, not at a party. I don't think you'll pull in these,' she says, smiling.

While the therapist is making my revolting little splints all I can think about is Seb. If he sees these will he run a mile? Forget the passion? Go off the sex? I'll have to hide them somewhere . . . in the wardrobe, under the bed?

The therapist is talking to me about protecting the hand and finger joints. I'm half listening, she's saying something about holding saucepans correctly. It's boring, practical. I never cook. Anyway, I am not going to have this rheumatoid arthritis for long so I don't need to worry. It will burn out, I reassure myself.

Two weeks after the diagnosis, I am clinging on to the hope that the rheumatoid arthritis will disappear, if not this autumn then next year. It has to. Friends are concerned. Rebecca, my old schoolfriend, comes round and asks whether the rumour is true – am I unwell? I tell her vaguely about the RA and that with any luck my body's just going through a weird phase, that's all. She hugs me warmly, saying she'll always be around if I need her.

'You're not going to America?' Seb asks incredulously.

'No, well, I'm not sure. If not this year next year,' I predict positively, as if nothing's really wrong. Why am I so calm, why aren't I crying, sobbing into his arms, telling him my plans are ruined? This weekend I am supposed to be signing the contract.

'At least it means I might have you around for longer. I'd miss you if you went,' he says. I don't think he knows what else to say. I don't want to talk about it.

I curl up in his lap watching the video *The Hand That Rocks the Cradle*. Seb holds my hand.

The film ends. I want to be close to Seb. We hug all night, my tears falling silently on his chest.

The therapist's voice is haunting me. 'You must wear the splints from day one, day one . . .'

I wait until Seb is fast asleep. Then I reach underneath the bed and quietly unfasten the Velcro.

19

Initial Reactions

'It's the devil playing games,' says Tom. 'Playing games with my sister. It's evil. It's wrong. Why not pick on someone who deserves it? I'll find out the answers for you when I'm in heaven.'

'You're not going to heaven quite yet though, are you?' I ask, watching him pace up and down the kitchen, dressed in his Nottingham Forest sweatshirt and scarf.

'No, I need to be here to look after you,' he says earnestly. 'We'll go to heaven together.' He pats my hand and kisses me clumsily on the cheek. 'You're my friend,' he says. I am close to tears.

Andrew is shy, sensitive, intelligent. He cannot express his feelings. Illness of any kind scares him. He hovers around me, humming and taking deep breaths. I know he is aching to say how sorry he is but the words just won't flow. I should help him out but I can't deal with it.

'What do you mean there's no cure? Why don't they know the cause? What can the doctors do?' Helen asks. Thank God Helen is home. She is just the person I need around. She keeps on playing with her green and gold ring. 'This is a temporary thing, Ali, you might have to spend a year resting but America's not to be given up on, no way. It's a fucking pain, but it'll be fine, just fine, sweetheart.' She kisses me on the forehead. I soak up the strength of her words.

Dad is very quiet.

Let me wake up soon. Come on, the joke's over. For the hundredth time I look at my right arm. This is my right arm, my right hand with which I serve at ninety miles per hour, hit backhand cross-court winners, pick up trophies. This hand is my future.

I cannot bear to tell any of my tennis friends. When I told Coach Peterson I felt ashamed and embarrassed. Arthritis is so unglamorous. I have this picture in my head of old, hunched ladies, not someone young like me.

Mum wrote to Peter, informing him of the recent diagnosis, and telling him I would no longer be able to play for the South Region. I wonder how he'll react?

But worst of all there is Bill. How am I going to tell him? He knows I have not been feeling well but he does not know about my visits to Casualty. He won't believe I have something like this.

'You must tell him,' Mum urged. 'I'll come with you, I want to talk to him anyway.'

'No,' I replied sharply. 'I don't need constant hand-holding. I am going to see him on my own after college today.'

I am counting my footsteps as I walk to the tennis club. I see the familiar sight of Bill's red car parked outside Court Five. My insides are knotted up, tangled like a plate of spaghetti. I think he's seen me, he's mouthing something in my direction. I could pretend I'm some dotty person wearing a Walkman, ignore him, and go home, but he starts to wave at me.

'Hi, how are you? Feeling better?' he asks.

'Yes,' I say instinctively. It's an innate response to say 'Yes, I'm fine' when you really mean 'Bloody awful.'

He opens the boot of the car and we both sit down on the edge.

'I mean no, actually I need to talk to you,' I stammer.

'Sure, fire away.' He is scribbling something in his appointments diary. I don't feel that I have his full attention. He highlights a date with his yellow marker.

'Bill, please.'

He closes the book. 'Sorry, all yours now,' he says, with a cheeky smile.

'You know I haven't been feeling well the last couple of months, well, I didn't know what it could be . . .' Alice, stop being so long-winded, just come out with it. 'Anyway, I have been to the doctor now and I have been told that I have something called rheumatoid arthritis. I don't know if you know anything about it, but it's to do with the joints.' There's a long, awkward pause. Say something please.

Eventually. 'I don't believe it,' Bill says quietly. He won't look at me.

'I was diagnosed two weeks ago, I would have told you earlier but . . .'

'No,' he explodes, 'there's no way a top athlete like you can have something like this. Who did you see?' he snaps angrily. 'They must have got it wrong. Have you had a second opinion?'

'No.'

'Doctors aren't perfect, infallible. They don't know you. I know you. This is crazy, you've got to see someone else.'

'I could do I suppose,' I say, shaking my head in agreement.

'I'm no doctor but I know you haven't got rheumatoid arthritis. You can't have.' He gets up and leans against the fencing of the tennis court, back turned towards me, gripping his hands tightly around the wire. I stand up, not knowing where to put my feet, or what to say. Bill turns round, slams the boot door down and sits behind the wheel. I long for him to say something reassuring. He opens his window. 'You see someone else,' he insists firmly, turns the engine on and grinds the car into gear. I watch him drive off into the distance at full speed, wondering what could be going through his mind.

I don't want to go into the clubhouse. I will bump into someone I know. I don't want to tell anyone else. Why was Bill so angry? Why couldn't he have hugged me, told me that everything would be all right? Perhaps there's no reason to comfort me. Bill's right, Dr Buckley could be wrong. I can't have rheumatoid arthritis.

I turn to walk home, but find myself walking back, through the gate and on to Court Five. I remember the gruelling practices Bill put me through before important tournaments and all the fun we've had together over the previous five years on this court. 'I'll soon be playing again,' I say, touching the net. 'Nothing's going to stop me. Nothing.'

It is the beginning of May. I am popping painkillers every four to six hours and sleeping badly. I feel lethargic – no energy. A levels in June and July are creeping up too quickly. Somebody press pause please. I have decided not to defer my A levels. I don't want life moving backwards. I have to take them.

I am not going to be left behind.

Medical Update:
Dr Buckley has prescribed Drug number 2 — indomethacin. This is one of the non-steroidal anti-inflammatory drugs (NSAIDs). He tells me it should relieve stiffness, inflammation and pain. I can hardly pronounce the names of these drugs but just hope they work.

20

King Lear

I have had rheumatoid arthritis for six weeks and the pain is getting worse.

Mum now sleeps with me in my bedroom. At night I hurt. My body is locked in one position. I feel as if I am superglued to my mattress, hammered down on to the sheets. I turn from one shoulder to the other. 'Mum, I'm sore, I'm sore,' I groan.

The deep and nagging pain, all over my body, seems eternal. With each tear I pray to see the morning. How can the change be so dramatic in only six weeks? Why am I feeling like this? Mum and I do some deep breathing exercises. Eventually, in the early hours of the morning, I drift off to the sound of Mum's Enya CD.

'Alice, call for you,' shouts Dad. 'It's Seb.'

I try to move off the sofa. I put one foot down and pain shoots up my leg. I wince. 'I can't move,' I say desperately, 'I can't move, Dad, look at me, what's happening?'

Dad rushes over, tears welling up in his eyes. 'Sod it,' he curses under his breath. He calls Mum.

'Can I come round and see her?' Seb asks. 'I want to see her.'

Seb is finding it hard to take in. I know he wants to be with me. He wants to help and support me. But . . .

'She can't come to the phone,' Dad says flustered. 'Call her tomorrow.' He hangs up abruptly and calls the GP on night duty.

The phone rings again. It's Granny wanting to talk to Mum.

'Is Alice not good?' she asks, immediately sensing something's wrong.

'No, she's in a lot of pain,' Mum replies.

Granny has seen and nursed terrible illnesses of all kinds while living in Africa, including once having to sew on a native boy's fingers which were mangled in a piece of farm machinery. Grandpa had very bad arthritis in his hips and her brother had rheumatoid arthritis. She is no stranger to pain.

'Please don't worry, Mum, we have the duty doctor coming out any moment. He'll be able to help Alice.'

However much Mum tries to reassure, she knows she has left Granny in a state of anxiety, feeling helpless on the other end of the line.

The doctor arrives. He prescribes a stronger painkiller and a sleeping pill. 'She ought to be in hospital,' he says.

The following morning Dr Buckley tells me I must be admitted into hospital straight away. Seb and Mum drive me. I'm not happy about it at all.

We enter the ward. It is a mixed rheumatology and surgical ward. The sight of old men snoring with tubes stuck into their bodies makes me feel so depressed. I can see an old man with a catheter sitting on his chair, his mouth wide open, dribble running down his cheek. A nurse tells me I am in the bed next to him.

'I am not sleeping there,' I shriek, quickly looking at Mum for back-up. 'Please,' I plead, 'can't I have a room of my own?' The nurse looks doubtful. 'I have revision,

I can't concentrate if I'm distracted. I must have a room of my own,' I insist.

Seb is sitting awkwardly on my bed. He tells me he has to leave. We walk to the lift. As the silver doors are about to meet he steps out again and holds me, kisses me as if it were our last meeting. 'I miss you already,' he whispers into my ear.

I walk slowly back to my room. Mum is unpacking my bag.

It's eight o'clock. I'm on my own. I feel alone. But at least I am not in a ward of wheezing old men.

One of the nurses knocks on the door. 'Hi, I'm Susie, I'll be looking after you,' she says chirpily.

'I don't want to be here. How long will I be here?' I demand.

'Hospitals aren't bad places. I'm sure you'll feel better when you leave. Now, just a few questions and then I'll leave you to get some sleep.'

It's so early. I can't close my eyes yet. I change into a new pair of pyjamas – the top has little teddy bears on it and says 'Peek a boo, I love you.' I lie on my bed and feel the crackle of the plastic mattress. 8.46 p.m. I feel restless. I play with the television remote control. Some stupid quiz show is on, wildlife on another channel. I can hear the ticking of the clock. I feel as if I have years of empty time ahead of me. 8.54 p.m. Time is an enemy, drawing everything out. What am I going to do? I put my Walkman on, and listen to 'Crowded House'. The night-time tea-trolley rattles around at ten and I steal five Rich Tea biscuits from the plate when the nurse's back is turned. Might as well eat, I have nothing else to do. 10.05 p.m. I'm lying awake thinking horrible things – A levels are in four weeks, I'll fail with two Us and an N, my friends will go off to college while I'm retaking, Seb will dump me because he hates hospitals and doesn't want a sick girlfriend, I'll be left behind, on the shelf like the Queen of Spades that nobody wants – the old maid. I have to do well in my exams. Suddenly passing my A levels has become one of the most important things in my life.

The following evening Dad is sitting at my bedside. He bought me some freesias on the way here which make my room smell nice. All the wards could do with some. I feel no different since taking indomethacin. Maybe it takes a little while to work, to get into my system? He opens his copy of *King Lear*, which I am studying for my English A level. He begins to recite his favourite passage, hand on heart.

'Why should a dog, a horse, a rat, have life and thou no breath at all . . .' he says woefully. 'Never, never, never, never, NEVER!' his voice rises. 'Do you see this? Look on her, look, her lips, look there, look there!'

'Carry on,' I say. 'My eyes are shut but I promise I'm listening.' Dad loves Shakespeare and would love to spend dreamy afternoons reading *Romeo and Juliet* or *Antony and Cleopatra* to Mum on grassy lawns with the birds singing and the picnic basket laden with crusty rolls, duck pâté, Brie, fruit cake and champagne, Mum's head on his shoulder lapping up every word. But Mum hates Shakespeare. So being in hospital with me is the next best thing for him. He flicks the pages and finds another favourite passage.

There's a knock on the door. 'Hi,' Bill says, opening the door tentatively. Dad slips out discreetly, saying he wants a cup of tea.

'I've been a fool, hardly supportive. I just didn't want to believe it,' Bill begins after an embarrassing silence. I have never seen Bill away from a tennis court. It feels strange talking to him in these surroundings. 'I know,' I say.

Bill is still hovering near the door. He sits down next to me. 'I'm sorry.' There's another long pause. 'Can they help you?' he asks.

'Yes. Well, I hope so.'

'I won't forget the fun we had on court. You really made it, whatever happens. You were . . .'

'Don't talk like that, in the past tense, as if it's all over.' I shift uneasily against the plastic pillows. 'I will play again, this will burn out,' I tell him forcefully.

His eyes are watering. He gets up and turns his back on me while he wipes his tears.

'Don't give up on me, Bill. I will get better.'

He turns and half smiles. 'Use the determination you had on the tennis court to beat this. I know you can.' He quickly kisses my forehead and leaves.

I feel invaded by sadness. Why do I feel like I won't see Bill again for a very long time? Surely this can't be the end?

Sophie visits me that evening bringing magazines. She holds my hand and listens to my depressing news. She wants me to go to Cornwall with her, her boyfriend, the rest of his family and Seb. I go to bed clutching on to the idea of a holiday, it's something to look forward to. And again I think of Bill and what he said to me.

It's my fifth day in hospital and I feel no different on the indomethacin. If anything the pain is worse. And despite the rest, my left knee has flared up. I have now learnt that when a joint or a number of joints are swollen and hot, causing pain and serious discomfort, this is called a flare-up. My knee feels like a little radiator, the fluid is bubbling like a stew. 'Where does this fluid come from?' I ask Dr Buckley, staring at my knee in disbelief.

'The synovial membrane, which lines the joint, becomes inflamed and that is what makes the joint so stiff and painful. Sometimes it goes no further than this. But in your case, fluid and cells have leaked out of the inflamed membrane. If we can extract the fluid, it will make the knee more comfortable for you. I'm also going to inject some steroid into the joint and this is very effective in reducing inflammation – it's the usual treatment for flare-ups like this.' He begins to get out the necessary equipment while I try to make sense of his words. Words which are familiar to him are another language to me. 'Tell me if I hurt you too much and I'll stop immediately,' he promises. He touches the knee, working out the best place to insert the needle that will draw out the fluid. It is a fat needle with a test tube and is truly terrifying. 'Now, think of somewhere nice and try to relax.'

My body is as taut as violin strings. I can't think of anything nice. OK, I'm running on a sandy beach with Seb, the water is clear blue . . .

The needle plunges in.

I breathe deeply. I am swimming with dolphins. Forget it. 'It hurts . . . FUCK, Oh God.' I squeeze the nurse's hand hard. 'Have you nearly finished?' I draw in a sharp breath.

'You're doing really well, good girl. So, you're reading *King Lear* I see,' Dr Buckley attempts, glancing at my book.

'Yes,' I whimper half-heartedly. I look down and can

see disgusting-looking, thick, yellow-orangey muck collecting in the tube.

'That's the one with Goneril and Regan isn't it? The silly fool gives up his kingdom . . .'

'Is it nearly over?' I ask, frowning. 'This is horrible . . . horrible.' The needle hits a particularly sensitive spot where the inflammation must be acute.

'Just a little more. There, now the steroid. There we go, all over.' He takes a plaster, draws a Mickey Mouse face on to it and sticks it on to my knee. 'Brave girl. That ought to give you some relief.' He sits for a few minutes trying to comfort me. 'You must get through your A levels, this will help. I'll come and see you tomorrow,' he says, leaving at last.

I lean back into my pillow and cry. What is happening to me?

I am sitting my first English paper, a four-hour exam, at our kitchen table. I'm relieved not to be in a crowded hall, sitting at a wooden, wobbly desk with paper jammed under one leg. One of the college tutors, Mr Barry, is sitting on our brown squeegee sofa in the corner of the room. He tells me to start. Please be something I've revised, I pray desperately. I turn the paper over, my fingers trembling. Part 1 involves answering a question related to a specific scene in *King Lear*. It is the passage where Lear is reconciled with Cordelia. Hurray, Dad read this out to me in hospital, he must have X-ray vision!

One hour into the exam and I have finished Part 1. My hands are throbbing and my knuckles look like red marbles. I rub them while skimming over Part 2, the choice of essay questions. I have to write two to complete the exam. It's OK, I still have plenty of time. The first one I choose is about the relationship of Edmund, the bastard son, with his father, Gloucester.

'Remember, take your breaks, Alice,' Mr Barry advises, when he sees me holding my sore hands. 'That's what the extra time's for.' I sit back and rest for a minute.

I'm working on the last essay and my hands feel as though they are about to drop off. I must try to finish, but I have only five minutes left.

Finally, Mr Barry tells me to put my pen down. I scribble down the last word and my inky pen stabs the full stop. As he gathers my papers poor Mr Barry's stomach growls. Mum and I hadn't thought of giving him any biscuits or drinks throughout the four hours. Oops.

After the exam Mum tells me to go to bed immediately and lie down. I take my Spanish folder with me, ready for Exam Number 2 tomorrow. There is no time to rest, I think irritably.

Later in the evening, Mum sends Tom up to tell me it's time for supper. He finds me asleep with my folder lying on top of me and A4 paper strewn over the bed. He tells Mum he didn't want to wake me. 'Does that mean I can have two extra sausages?' he asks hopefully.

It's the morning of my Spanish exam and my right knee is the size of a balloon, a melon even. Another flare-up. I ring Dr Buckley in a panic. He says he'll see me immediately at the hospital. He extracts the gunge and gives me another steroid injection to reduce the inflammation.

'Good luck for this afternoon,' he says, 'I'm crossing my fingers for you. If you don't know it now . . .'

'You'll never know it,' I shrug.

*

My remaining exams follow a similar pattern. I see Dr Buckley in between each one and he extracts fluid from my writing hand, or injects painful knees. Each time I see him, he continues drawing a Mickey Mouse face on the plasters and winks, saying he's rooting for me. He's becoming a wonderful friend. I don't know how I'd have got through my exams without him.

A levels are over! Sophie, Seb and a few other friends drive over to my house and take me out to celebrate. I hope I never have to think about exams again. And we all hope I will soon begin to get better.

Medical Update:
Dr Buckley has prescribed Drug Number 3 – Methotrexate. 'Methotrexate is an anti-cancer as well as anti-rheumatic drug,' he tells me. A real treat, two gems rolled into one. 'It's much more aggressive, prescribed for the particularly difficult cases, patients who aren't getting enough relief from the NSAIDs. If it works it should prevent joint damage and slow down the disease process.' I am a difficult case. Oh well. At least I excel in something.

21

The Party

Wimbledon is on. Agassi is playing but I hardly recognize him because he's dressed immaculately in white and his hair's shorter. It's the quarter-finals against Becker, who is, as usual, diving and jumping around for the ball. Come on, Agassi. I watch intently for twenty minutes, wishing I was there.

It's two days after my last exam and I'm back in hospital, where they are monitoring me on my new drug.

A label is stuck to the head of my bed which reads 'On bedrest'. After four days in hospital my body feels like a heavy brick. I lie still all day, like a useless lump of wood, occasionally opening my mouth like a goldfish to receive the nurse's thermometer, or extending an arm for her to take my blood pressure. The only form of exercise I can do is hydrotherapy, which is lovely. The water is heated to 96 degrees and the physiotherapist goes through exercises with floats and rings. I feel as light as a butterfly in the water. I look forward to the mornings when my friendly grey-haired porter comes to take me down to the hot bath.

'Alice, have you just been to the loo on your own?' a nurse asks. I look guilty. 'You must ring your buzzer. Bedrest means bedrest, not getting up at all,' she says.

I am not going to have a plastic bedpan shoved underneath me every time I need to go. Who do they think they're dealing with? I must remember that now I'm a difficult case.

But I used to be a great prospect, with a junior world ranking and I was seeded at the Nationals. I was the girl with thirty offers from the USA, all of them wanting me. Charlotte is in America, hoping to fulfil her dreams. And where am I, where am I going? I am in a dreadful hospital and I'm going nowhere. I can't even go to the loo on my own.

Bill hasn't visited me again. Maybe he'll come soon. Why won't he come? I wish he would. Yet I want to blot people like Charlotte and Connie out of my life. Staying in touch with college friends like Sophie, Rebecca and Seb, who are not part of my tennis, is much easier.

It's Seb's eighteenth birthday party tomorrow night. I have got to go. I am not going to fester in here like a mouldy cabbage, imagining what a wonderful time my friends are all having without me. 'Can I go?' I beg Dr Buckley when he is doing his ward rounds. 'Seb will be so upset if I don't go.'

Dr Buckley, like a god, stands with his team of young student doctors and nurses. 'Concentrate on exercises first,' he says, looking amused. 'Can you put your hands behind your neck and on your head? . . . Can you clench your hand into a fist? . . . Does this hurt?' he queries, gently squeezing the knuckles on the hand. 'Does that feel tender?' he asks, bending and flexing my knees.

The student doctors are making notes on my range of movement. I find it hard to extend my arms fully, and I wish they'd stop gawping. I am not an exhibit. 'Can I go tomorrow? I promise I'll come straight back, I'm feeling so much better,' I lie desperately.

He raises an eyebrow. 'I shouldn't really let you go, you know, but I will. Have some fun,' he whispers.

'You can wind him round your little finger,' says the nurse after he's gone. 'All you need to do is flutter your eyelashes.' She shakes her head. She's probably jealous, I think smugly.

I'm scanning my wardrobe. What am I going to wear? I need something bright, something which says, 'I'm OK.' I pick out my short lime green dress with spaghetti straps which cross over at the back, revealing a lot of bare skin. Just the job. I do not want anyone to suspect anything. I don't want people to think I'm still in hospital. I'm just going to go out and have a good time like everyone else.

Tom comes into my room when I'm half dressed and quickly turns round, banging his head into my door. 'Sorry, thought you were ready, how much for the gun,' he mutters, stumbling out of my room. My brother is beginning to pick up odd expressions. He's four years older than me but I feel as if he's my younger brother. We're all worried about him. We know he has never been one hundred per cent normal since birth but it's more complex than that. Yet no doctor can diagnose exactly what's wrong with him.

'Tom, don't go. Entertain me with some jokes,' I say. 'I'm dressed now. Or put some music on, I need to get in the mood.' I begin to put on my make-up, taking much more care than usual. Tom puts a James Bond soundtrack on and dances around my room with a towel draped across his shoulders. 'The man with the golden gun,' he sings, making me smile. He looks at me, 'Bond, James Bond, shaken not stirred,' he says and then howls with laughter.

*

I walk into a crowded, smoky bar but luckily spot Sophie immediately. She squeezes my hand and squeals, 'I'm so glad you could come! Let's get a drink.' She's drunk already. I have not seen Seb yet, I search the crowds but cannot find him. 'Hey you!' Sophie's boyfriend says to me from behind. I swing round and give him a hug. 'Come and dance.' Why not, who cares if my knees hurt, alcohol will numb the pain. I'm going to forget all about it tonight. I take a big gulp of my drink and follow him on to the dance floor. As the previous song fades out, the DJ dedicates the next song to me from Seb: UB40, 'Red, Red Wine'. I look around and eventually spot him at the bar, his friendly face smiling down at me.

After a couple of songs I have had enough, I go back up to the bar. My feet are aching. I start thinking about the following morning, going back to hospital. 'Stop it,' I think, pinching myself. Someone from college comes up and asks me if I am better.

'Much,' I reply, smiling. 'I really am.'

'That's great,' he says. 'So you're still going to America?'

'Oh yes, definitely,' I reply, feeling positive. I have another couple of drinks. Life is great, I am young, I am going to play tennis again. Yes, life is wonderful. I go and join Sophie and Seb on the dance floor.

Later, tucked up in bed, I feel cosy and warm. I'm still the same old Alice, I think, curling up under the covers and drifting off to sleep. Life is rosy. Life is like lying peacefully in a field, bathed in warm sunlight and surrounded by beautiful sunflowers.

The following morning I feel terrible. I feel as if a double-decker bus has run over me in the night – and then decided to reverse too, just to make sure the damage was done. My eyes look black from rubbed-off mascara. I look as if I was in a fight the night before. I struggle to get out of bed and limp downstairs in my pyjamas. Mum is sewing. I make some coffee.

'How was the party?' Mum asks brightly.

'Fine.' I can only manage a monosyllabic reply. 'I might watch some TV,' I say eventually, sloping off into the playroom.

'Alice, you have to be back at the hospital this morning. I don't want to rush you, but you'll have to get going soon. They are expecting you back,' Mum reminds me nervously. I think she's scared of me. She thinks I'm a bomb that might explode at any time.

'Oh God,' I snap. The seconds are ticking. Blast off. 'I don't fucking want to go back. I won't go, you can't fucking make me go.' Reality dawns. I hate it.

After two and a half weeks in hospital, Dr Buckley says I can leave the next day. He injects steroid into my ankles, which look the size of golfballs, and into one of my elbows. The fluid is working overtime, leaking into every joint it can. I feel like a bruised pincushion.

That night Sophie visits me. 'Hi, let's go outside,' she says, walking awkwardly. She has a few cans of wine under her coat. She pushes me in a maroon-seated wheelchair, as I am still on bedrest. We go to the playground area where visitors and patients often sit, and pour the wine into plastic cups. We talk about the plans to go to Cornwall. It will be a proper holiday.

'I don't want to think about hospitals for a long, long time,' I say, gently pushing myself up and down on the swing. 'Can you believe all this has happened?'

'No, it still hasn't sunk in. You are going to get better,

Ali,' Sophie says, reaching out for my hand. 'We're all here for you, you can't get rid of me that easily.' She bites her lip; she always does that when she's being serious.

'I miss my tennis,' I say, looking down to the ground, my long hair falling loosely around my face. 'It's like losing a friend.'

'I know,' she responds quietly. 'I wish I'd watched you play in a proper match. I would have been so proud of you.'

Sophie pushes me back to the ward. We've lost track of time and it is now well past ten o'clock. The lights are dimmed, there is snoring. We try to be as quiet as possible and not bump into anything. Sophie crashes into the bedside table and all my pills clatter to the floor. We laugh hysterically.

'Alice, it's late, come on, bed,' one of the nurses orders, helping us pick up the pills. 'Your friend should have left ages ago.' The buzzers start ringing; somebody is farting on the commode. The nurse's back is turned. I look at Sophie. Take me home, back to your house for the night, I pray. I can discharge myself!

'Quick, let's get your things.' Sophie sounds like my mother, but then she is a motherly figure. 'Quick, before the nurse comes back.' I cheer up immediately and she pushes me out of the ward, my luggage on my lap. We are laughing. I'm free. I'm ready for a holiday.

I'm free.

Medical Update:
The methotrexate will take a while to 'kick in'. As a type of bridge therapy, Dr Buckley has prescribed Drug Number Four — a course of predniso-lone, a steroid. He tells me it is a miracle drug, reducing inflammation overnight. But long-term use can cause awful side-effects such as toxic-ity in the body, acne, weight gain, mood swings and thinning of the bones, leading to osteoporosis and fractures.

22

The Brown Envelope

The day of our A level results has finally come. Sophie is in Portugal; I am going into college with Seb to collect my brown envelope.

The common-room is buzzing.

'Read yours first,' Seb says.

'Why me? You can. I don't want us to open them here anyway,' I say, hearing both laughter and tears around me.

This little brown envelope is like a magic key to a door. I must step through it with my friends, I don't want to be left on the wrong side, still knocking. I grip it tightly. 'I can't open it here,' I repeat, tugging at his green rugby shirt, 'I won't.'

'Right, home then,' Seb grins, taking my hand, obviously far more relaxed than me.

Seb pulls over at an off-licence. 'We need something to celebrate with if we do well,' he says. 'Or to drown our sorrows,' he adds, kissing me through the window. His back turns.

I can't look at my envelope. I want to be back in Cornwall, away from it all. Spending a week with Seb was wonderful, the slight awkwardness between us vanished. We were a normal boyfriend and girlfriend again. Seb taught me to surf and was always ready to pick me up when the huge waves knocked me down. Sophie, with her long, wavy dark hair and blue and red wetsuit, looked like Wonderwoman. In the evenings, tired from surfing, Sophie and I left the boys on the beach and helped Maggie, Sophie's boyfriend's mother, cook the supper – with frequent gin and tonic and cigarette breaks in between! And the steroid drug is magic. I was able to go on long beach walks and even managed some rock-climbing, although afterwards my feet were twice the usual size. Sophie called them my 'magic feet' – in the morning they were small and by the evening, large.

We played drinking games. Sophie and I sprayed Maggie's Chanel No. 5 down the boys' boxer shorts one night and had to own up to it the following morning when she was wondering where her new expensive perfume had gone.

I felt like an ordinary, normal teenager again, although I kept moaning at Seb about my moon face, a side-effect from the steroid. 'My cheeks are fat,' I complained every morning. He squeezed them playfully and told me he loved my face. He gave me confidence and assured me I was not a burden when I was tired and needed piggy-backs. He told me I would get better soon, 'out of prison', he said, and free to do all the things I wanted again.

Seb rarely gets depressed, anxious or low – his cheery outlook on life makes me feel so much better. I am dreading the day he leaves. He plans to go travelling around New Zealand and Australia for six months in September. I feel like our time's running out.

I look down at my envelope. The suspense is too much. I rip it open.

English . . . B. French . . . B. Oh my God, this is fantastic, I've passed two out of three. Bs are OK. I turn over the sheet. Spanish . . . C. Well, I could have done better in that one but I've passed! I look at Seb's envelope and can't help opening it. He got an A in Graphics. He is walking back towards the car. I quickly put the envelope back on the dashboard. 'I got two Bs and a C,' I cry out. 'And you got an A in Graphics,' I add quickly.

'I can't believe you opened it,' he gasps incredulously, trying to sound put out, but his wide smile tells me I'm forgiven. Seb got an A, a B and a C. We put the music on loudly and drive home feeling very proud of ourselves. I keep leaning over to kiss Seb and he nearly drives into a ditch.

At home Mum opens some champagne. Seb puts his arm around me and we drink to the future, to us.

I ring Helen, I ring Dad at work.

I'm through the door. Today I feel happier than I have felt in a long time.

Medical update:
Dr Buckley prescribes Drug Number 5 – a powerful drug called sulphasalazine to back up the methotrexate. Apparently they are great friends, they make a delicious cocktail. 'But there are awful side-effects too,' he tells me. 'Nausea, abdominal pain, rashes, headaches, irritability, dizziness and bone marrow suppression.' I tell him I don't care, I'll take anything that might help. I collect the pills from Pharmacy – they are nasty, large, and yellow.

23

'The Cat Sat on the Mat'

'The cat sat on the mat,' I type. My silver bracelet jangles up and down. 'The cat sat on the mat.' I glance at the clock – 12.20 p.m. I feel an enormous lump in my throat; Seb's gone. I touch the bracelet again.

Seb gave it to me last night. He said he hoped things would be exactly the same when he got back, that we would still be together. I scribbled on a piece of paper how much I loved him, and gave him a photograph of myself. I don't want him forgetting what I look like. I have his face fixed in my mind. Blue eyes, soft blond hair, wide smile. Lying on his bed, I turned some music on and turned off the lights. I did not want him to see or hear me crying. But the pauses in between each song gave us away – we were both crying.

This morning, after saying goodbye to Seb again, I drove away in the rain, tears pouring down my cheeks. I almost drove into the back of a lorry, my vision was so distorted. I crawled along – a Mini Metro raced past me – to my secretarial course, looking at my watch constantly. Seb's flight was at 12.10 p.m.; he had a standby ticket. I suppose I was hoping there might be a chance he would not get a seat, but now he'll be watching a movie and eating a chunk of duty-free Toblerone. He'll be in the clouds, on his way to New Zealand, and he won't be back for at least six months.

Seb's been my lifeline. We've talked about the RA but our relationship hasn't changed, if anything it is stronger. I am happy for him that he's gone. He gets restless and he loves travelling. But I feel empty and deeply insecure, I'm terrified it's going to be, 'out of sight, out of mind'. And, selfishly, I cannot help thinking, 'You're leaving just when I need you the most.' When Seb walked out of the door, I wanted to shout after him, 'Take me with you, wait for me.'

'The cat sat on the mat.' As I type the line for the fifth time, I am confronted with the reality of my situation: this last summer, being diagnosed, my time in hospital – it isn't an awful dream, it's real. For the first time I feel as if the door has been shut in my face.

Miss Sprules, the secretarial course, is the last thing I want to be doing. 'But it's better than doing nothing, everybody needs to know how to type these days,' Mum said – not me though, I should be in America, meeting new coaches, meeting new players, flying from one tournament to another. People should be telling me they love my accent. I should not be here.

By some miracle Rebecca is on the course too. Her travel plans have been put on hold and she clinched the last Miss Sprules place. We sit next to each other in a room of about twelve other girls – it's like being back at school. The girls all look so dreary to me, with their velvet hairbands and white frilly blouses. Why do I have to be with these people?

Sprules is strict, trousers cannot be worn. Mum made me a tartan full-length skirt, maybe she thought it would help me fit in. I never wear it.

We have two teachers, word-processing in the morning, typing in the afternoon. The head teacher at Sprules, Miss Murray, is very kind and organized some part-time work for me at a small commercial contracting firm soon after my course began. I am happy to divide my day and earn some money. I hope I might begin to feel better soon and be able to join Seb for a while. I am going to start saving. Miss Murray asked me whether I wanted to let the company know about my condition but I said no. I don't want anyone to know.

I work mainly for the general manager, Richard, whose office is just behind my desk. He is young, tall, dark and good-looking. Every time he comes out of his office to dictate a letter to me I am terrified he will notice the lump on my wrist, which looks like a hard-boiled egg. And one of the middle knuckles on my right hand is tight and swollen. It looks as if a marble is bursting out of it.

It's mid October and the autumn leaves are changing colour. I'm staring at the clock. Four p.m. I'm at work but everything has flared up. I should not have struggled in today, sometimes I'm so stupid. Underneath my desk, I rub my knees. They seem to be on fire, I could toast marshmallows on them, or fry crispy bacon. They feel boggy, my kneecap is no longer prominent but lost in the thick fluid. Luckily I am wearing a long grey skirt – gone are the days of my lime green mini-dresses.

Richard comes out and plonks some paper on my desk. 'Hi, these need photocopying quickly. I've got a meeting in half an hour.' The photocopier is downstairs. Painfully, I stand up. Ten minutes later I walk into his office with the duplicated copies.

'Sorry, I forgot to give you these too,' he says, giving me a couple more sheets. 'And can you speed up? I'm running late.'

I feel as though my legs are about to collapse and the fluid tightens at every bend.

Five thirty comes. The post has been franked and collected.

'Shit, have I missed the post?' Sharon from downstairs asks, out of breath. 'I have to get this letter off.' She looks at me, her expression like a puppy-dog wanting a bone.

'We can still catch it,' I say, taking the letter from her.

'Can you? Thanks, you're brilliant.'

A doormat more like. I get my coat and walk down the road, letter in hand. My feet are telling me angrily that they have had enough. I am dreaming about soaking them in hot water, letting the pain evaporate into the frothy bubbles. I reach the postbox and turn round, seeing the long stretch of pavement ahead of me. Tears of frustration run down my face. Will somebody please invent a machine which takes me where I want to be at the touch of a button? Of course, if I did have one of those, I wouldn't be here, I'd be with Seb in New Zealand.

I am determined not to tell any of the people at the company about my problems. I do not want sympathy, I do not want to be treated differently. Covering up is an art at which I have become very good.

My life follows this thrilling routine for a couple more weeks – Sprules, work, home, *EastEnders* and bed.

Life at home is terrible. Tom's mood swings become much worse. It is clear he is unable to hold down a job, especially as Tom's doctor has finally diagnosed mild schizophrenia. Mum and Dad are devastated, although his diagnosis does not come as a surprise. They are desperately trying to get him settled into a community for the mentally handicapped in Wales. My being at home does not help him. One side of Tom is extremely affectionate but the other is insanely jealous of the attention I receive – first with the tennis, now with my RA. Tom is a worry to my parents, his future is uncertain. I wish I was distanced from his situation. I have no patience with him and I don't understand how anyone can be jealous of me now.

Sophie, more than anyone, keeps me going. She is going to Romania to work in an orphanage, but not until after Christmas. She often comes round in the evening for supper, or we go to the cinema. She has accepted a place at Bristol University for the following autumn.

Things begin to get worse. I walk to work one afternoon, feeling queasy. The revolting yellow pill I swallow every morning is not helping, it only makes me feel sick. I arrive, relieved to be able to sit down. I notice some letters and menus on my desk which need to be typed. I can hear Richard on the phone next door. I look at the piece of paper on top of the pile. The letters start swirling around, they are blurred. Saliva is bubbling in my mouth, I rush to the loo to spit it out. I lock myself in and sit down. I feel drunk, my vision is blurring, I shut my eyes and feel as if I'm on a fair ride. It's the waltzer and a horrible man keeps spinning me round and round. I hear footsteps.

Richard knocks on the door. 'Alice, are you all right? You've been in there for ages, it's just that I need to go,' he says.

I want to be swallowed up right now. I unlock the door.

'I'm feeling a bit sick, I don't know why it's suddenly come on.' Illness shame. Almost an affliction in itself.

'Must have been a late night,' he jokes. If only. I have not been to a party for ages.

'Do you mind if I go home? I don't think I'll be much use today,' I say.

I am in Dr Buckley's office, waiting for him to come back. During my appointment he was summoned urgently to the ward. I peer at my folder. Confidential is stamped on the outside. Well, it is me. What have they got to hide? I pick up the folder and a letter falls out.

'. . . Alice is a pleasant girl who doesn't drink or smoke . . . thirty per cent of people who get arthritis recover completely within a few years.'

I'm sure that's me. Mine will burn out. I continue to read.

'Sixty per cent continue to have flare-ups with pain and difficulty, but can lead close to a normal life.' Not me.

'But this unfortunate girl, I fear, is in the last group, the ten per cent bracket, whose rheumatoid arthritis is so severe it will lead to disability . . .'

My heart stops. I read it again. I shove the letter back inside. I don't want to see Dr Buckley. I pick up my bag and leave the office. The waiting-room is filled with depressing figures – a lady with a walking stick, a man in a wheelchair, a mother with a baby in splints. I don't want to be part of this. I walk straight past them all, down the corridor, out of the ward. I should not be here. I'm terrified.

'We already knew,' Dad confesses quietly, when I tell him about the letter.

'Well, thanks for telling *me*,' I shout.

'It was just before A levels, we couldn't have told you then. We probably should have, I don't know,' he says, shaking his head in distress.

'Unfortunate girl. Pain. Disability. That's not me,' I say, boiling with rage. 'How can they know this already? How can they be so sure? I am not pleasant, I hate that word. And I do drink and I've started smoking. See, they don't know a bloody thing.'

'Alice, calm down,' Mum orders firmly. 'We did what we thought best at the time.'

'Calm down?! Why should I?' I shout in exasperation. 'You should have told me!' I storm out of the room, slamming the door shut behind me.

I need to follow a different path.

I won't let that be me.

24

Cider Vinegar and Honey

Friends keep sending Mum and me information about alternative therapies, healers, dieticians . . .

'Have you tried coral calcium? It's collected from a coral reef around the Japanese islands of Okinanawa and Tocunoshima,' says one.

'My grandfather has arthritis in his thumb and a nutritionist put him on to a diet of nothing but raw vegetables.'

'You must go and see Mo-Mo, the Yugoslavian healer. He flicks his wrist over you to unblock the energy . . .'

'Pull your fillings out, your teeth out if necessary. It's the mercury poisoning you. I know a super man who'll do it for you . . .'

'My husband has arthritis and stings himself with bees, the poison works wonders.'

'Granny bathes in Dead Sea salts, you can buy them from Boots.'

'Have you ever thought about seeing a spiritual healer? Or going to healing services in church?'

'Have you tried "stress and anxiety" tablets? You take up to six a day . . .'

'Celery pills are the answer.'

'Magnets work.'

Soon I am rushing around like a headless chicken, trying to find the most obscure pills and cures. I don't want to take pills which do nothing but make me feel sick. I've got to find something else which will help, I think determinedly.

'Hello, my name's Albert.'

He is a funny-looking man. He looks as though he is kitted out in Oxfam clothes — he is wearing a brown diamond-patterned jumper, light grey flared trousers and comfortable-looking Clarks shoes. There is an awkward silence. The church is now empty. 'I couldn't help noticing the way you walked up to the front,' he says to me eventually. He has a squashed-up face, pinched little blue eyes and a button mouth. 'I am a healer myself. Why did you come here?'

'I have rheumatoid arthritis.' I begin to feel more interested.

'It's terrible, unbelievable,' Sophie adds. 'She used to be a tennis player but her RA is so bad she can't play any more.'

'You are lucky to have such a supportive friend,' Albert smiles. Thin little pursed lips open, revealing nicotine-stained teeth. 'I can tell you two are very close, am I right?'

We nod.

'I've done a lot of healing in my time and had a lot of success. If you're interested . . .'

That night Sophie and I talk about it. Is he genuine, have I got anything to lose?

Albert is sitting at the corner table of the restaurant with a paper and coffee. He is still wearing the patterned jumper and grey trousers. He talks about himself. He has been a successful journalist, he has always been dedicated to the Church. He believes he has healing powers. 'I was on a retreat in Lourdes . . .'

'Where Our Lady is supposed to have appeared,' steps in Sophie.

'Something mysterious happened. A stranger battled her way through the masses to get to me. She looked me straight in the eye and placed a ring on my finger.' He shows us the silver ring on his third finger. Flesh is bulging on either side, it is so tight. 'I have never been able to take it off since. I think that is a sign in itself, don't you? She told me I was blessed with remarkable healing powers,' he says. 'And,' he pauses, 'I have never been to Hampshire before. Something called me here, you understand. Do you see what I'm saying?'

Sophie and I arrange to see Albert again in a few days.

We are sitting in a smart hotel. Sophie and I wonder how he can afford to live in such luxury, judging by his tattered clothes.

'I told the staff that I would be seeing two pretty young girls here and that it's nothing sexual,' Albert twitches. 'I don't want anyone getting the wrong ideas, you see. You know how people can gossip.'

Sophie and I stare at him.

'Healing is all about accepting,' he begins. He darts off to the reception desk and comes back, out of breath. 'If I try desperately to aim this piece of paper into the bin I can guarantee it won't go in.' He scrunches the piece of paper up and throws it towards the bin. 'You see,' he smiles, picking it up off the floor. 'Now, if I throw this piece of paper without trying it will land straight in.' He throws it over his shoulder. 'See.'

'It didn't go in actually,' I say.

'It's never not worked,' he exclaims. 'But you under-stand my theory? You understand?'

Sophie and I both nod vigorously.

Albert organizes an 'all night prayer session'. He rings up his friends, telling them to think of me on the same night. 'Everyone praying for you all over the country is extremely powerful,' he says.

Weird though it may seem, I am feeling better. Perhaps it's psychosomatic, I don't know. But I want to carry on seeing him and Sophie comes with me, although she reminds me it's nothing sexual.

Albert complains of a sore finger and asks me to say a prayer for him. 'As friends now, I'm asking you to help. I'm going through a rough time,' he tells us. Sophie is trying not to laugh as she looks into my speechless face.

He is becoming obsessed, following me around. I feel as if he is now depending on me. I meet him in a hotel bar. Sophie is away so I am on my own, but I am going to tell him that our 'friendship' has to end.

Albert takes large gulps of his drink and keeps slam-ming his glass on to the table as if to make a point. 'But I had so many ideas for you, you understand.'

'I can't see you any more,' I repeat. Both Sophie and I decided we had to put an end to this, that we could not see him any more. I just wish she was with me to tell him too. Suddenly that twitchy smile is irritating me. He follows me to my car. I feel scared for the first time. I lock the door immediately, my hand shaking. The car won't start. He bangs on the window. I steady my hand and the engine finally comes to life. I breathe in deeply and drive away.

*

The phone rings at home the following afternoon. 'Hello. Do you know a man called Albert Skinner?' asks the owner of the hotel where Albert and I last met.

'Yes. Why?'

'He has left our hotel, running up a huge bill, without paying. His bedroom is in a state. We saw from his phone bill that he called you. Do you know where your friend is?'

'No,' I reply, shocked.

I never see him again.

I feel let down. Disappointed. Gullible. Naïve. But I don't regret meeting him. I have to take chances, it could have worked. Strange things happen. So, come on. What can I try next?

A relative makes it her mission to cure me. She advises me to spit on a piece of paper and fold it into four pieces to send to a doctor in Scotland – apparently a lot can be told from your saliva. The doctor rings up and asks me whether my childhood was happy and did I have bad dreams? I hang up immediately. Her second suggestion is to drink lots of cider vinegar and honey. And suggestion number three: 'There is a book,' she says, written by Elizabeth Beckett, who claims she can 'cure' arthritis with a special diet among many other things. 'Cure' has become a magic word. Since I am getting little benefit from the drugs, Mum is just as keen as me to give this a try. We decide to go and visit her at a clinic in Shropshire. Dad is cynical.

We are sitting in the waiting-room. The door to her room opens slowly and there she stands, a slender vision in white. She looks very young. She ushers us in and asks us to sit down. She talks very slowly and clearly. At first she wants to know a little about me, then I have a blood pressure test which is so low the machine is accused of being faulty. Her major concern is the drugs I am taking, as she is worried about their strength, their toxicity and the possible long-term side-effects. If I start the treatment and it proves effective, she hopes I might be able to reduce my drug intake and gradually wean myself off them. Her treatment involves a strict diet avoiding caffeine and acids, bathing joints in special oils and Epsom Salts, taking vitamin and mineral supplements and drinking fungi tea. 'The vast majority of my patients feel better in themselves after six weeks. You must let the body heal itself. You must not come off your drugs yet, but try not to resort to the steroid injections which only mask the pain.' There is a pause. 'I have helped so many people, and I can cure you,' she says. 'If you persevere I believe you will get better.'

'You really think you can help?' I ask. I hardly dare look at Mum.

'Yes,' she says emphatically. 'I know I can.'

25

A Day in the Life of an Alternative Freak

At breakfast, I open my box of vitamins and minerals. Each type is sealed in a separate clear plastic bag. Out pop folic acid, magnesium, Vitamin A, Vitamin B, which has a huge family – B complex, B1, B2, B3, B6, B12; Vitamin D, Vitamin K, zinc, Vitamin C with rosehip, pantothenic acid, kelp, iron, alfalfa – the list is endless. I arrange the rainbow-coloured pills around my glass of bottled Evian water; they look like pretty beads.

Each pill I swallow smells worse than the one before. Pill number 12, multi-vitamin. In it goes. It stinks of dog biscuits. Yuck. I swish down yet more Evian water to take the taste away.

Tom comes into the kitchen, dressed in his shoes, cap and purple dressing-gown. 'How are your legs?' he asks.

'Terrible.'

'Well, we all die,' he says cheerfully and puts the kettle on.

Tom and I are becoming close. I am trying to understand how his muddled mind works. People are very ready to ask how I am, but no one dares to ask Mum and Dad about Tom, the quirky, misfit child. It hurts him. He hates being in the shadow of people's lives, always feeling the odd one out. But now he can relate to my fears and disappointments and the physical limitations which come with the RA.

'I'd buy you a new body if I could,' he says earnestly.

'And I'd give you a new brain.'

'I'd like that, a new brain for Thomas.'

I ask him to help me make my fungi tea. Tom wrinkles up his nose, telling me it looks disgusting. 'It looks more like slimy jellyfish,' he says. I tell him irritably that people are all too ready to swallow pills full of chemicals, pills of unknown origin, but when it comes to natural concoctions we are peculiarly sceptical.

'I'd rather have a pill, I think,' he says.

Molasses, full of iron, and a laxative, helps to prevent anaemia – but is truly disgusting. I hold my nose and eat two teaspoons of the brown gooey gunge.

Tom hands me a cup of tea. 'The devil's broth, m'lady,' he says darkly. 'To drink with the devil's food.'

We prepare a bowl of hot water with Epsom Salts to dunk my feet into. Epsom salts help to remove acids from the body. Tom walks towards me; the water is swilling around and little puddles are forming on the floor.

I brush my teeth three times before going to work. I know my breath smells. Last weekend Helen kissed me good morning and then immediately shied away. 'Alice, is fungus growing in your mouth?' she asked.

I make my acid-free packed lunch to take to work – raw vegetable salad with wholemeal bread and a banana. Elizabeth Beckett says nettle tea is wonderful and soon I won't want to drink anything else. I pop a couple of nettle tea sachets into my bag.

Richard is in a good mood, he tells us he is going to buy everyone in the office a treat. He comes back with cream cakes filled with acidic strawberries for tea. I look at mine longingly. 'Acid' is ringing in my ears but my mouth is watering. Elizabeth said, 'Stay well clear of anything that makes your mouth water as it's bound to be acidic.' But I really want to eat it, dammit.

'Well, aren't you going to eat it?' he asks.

'Oh yes, in a minute, it looks delicious,' I gush.

The minute Richard goes back into his office, I go to the loo and wrap the cake up in tissue paper to take home, as I know Dad will enjoy it. When he reappears, I pretend how lovely it was, licking my lips.

Once back from work, I set up my bowl of warm water with lavender oil, which is meant to have healing properties, and soak my feet while watching television and drinking another cup of scrumptious nettle tea.

Mum calls out from the kitchen, 'Alice, you have the choice of black-eyed bean casserole or buckwheat and red lentil bake for supper.'

'Well, what do you want?'

'Oh no, we're having spaghetti bolognese.'

Dad opens a bottle of wine and I have to sprinkle some form of powder into my glass that Elizabeth gave me. It's supposed to get rid of the acid. I can't think how it works. Tom tells me the powder looks more like dandruff. He is fascinated by my diet. I look into my glass, and suddenly I've gone off drinking wine anyway.

I'm trying not to watch Dad eat his spaghetti. You are enjoying your black-eyed beans, I tell myself, but I can't eat it all. Mum gives the leftovers to Meggy, our Norwich terrier, whose lethal breath is on a par with mine. Mum has to brush her teeth twice a week with Colgate. Meggy leaves the beans untouched.

Before bedtime I soak in a hot bath. After the bath, I dry quickly and roll into bed, where I dream endlessly about chocolate, strawberries and cream.

26

Indecision

It's 1993, a New Year. Steffi Graf lost to the grunter, Monica Seles, in three sets at the Australian Open. Mum is making box-pleated lampshades, Helen is in love, I am still on my diet . . .

I am sick of wholemeal this, wholemeal that — I long for a chocolate bar, proper coffee, soft doughy WHITE bread, thick creamy mayonnaise, curried chicken and rhubarb crumble with toffee ice-cream.

I have been following this diet religiously for six weeks, doing everything by the book, but it's not been easy. I don't feel I'm getting anywhere. I haven't been able to reduce my intake of drugs and my body is crying out for a steroid fix. Do I feel a sense of well-being? No, I do not. I feel weak.

'I can't walk, Mum,' I say, trying to get out of the car.

Mum pulls me up from under the shoulders.

'No, I can't move,' I protest.

Fred, our friendly builder who is working on the out-side shed, asks if we need a hand.

'Do you think you could help, that would be so kind,' Mum thanks him shakily.

His strong arms carry me to the sitting-room.

'I'm not normally like this,' I murmur with shame, unable to look at him.

'You just rest, take it easy, love,' he says, and then turns away, fighting tears.

I ring Elizabeth Beckett, begging her to put me in touch with someone else who has been through this agony. During my first consultation, she read out a few letters to me from patients who had benefited from her treatment, so it should be easy for her to put me in touch with somebody. Elizabeth Beckett's assistant is unhelpful, though, and she does not pass on any names. Where is crippled Mr Dicker, the gardener, who previously couldn't walk, but is now up and down ladders all day pruning roses to his heart's content? And where is Mrs Pratt, who previously sat in her chair all day long but now dances through the night? And what about the fireman who had to give up his job but now drops down the poles at the speed of lightning? Where are they? Why can't I ring one of them up? Why isn't she helping me more? Encouragement, that's all I need.

I put the phone down and sit, frozen. I've made a terrible mistake, I'm gullible, she's laughing behind my back. She's a complete fraud. She's only in it for the money. I can see her counting my pound coins and arranging my five pound notes in tall piles. I can see her packaging dog biscuits into little boxes and laughing as she labels them 'Vitamin C with Rosehip'. I'm giving up. Look at me, I can't even walk. I want to be back with Dr Buckley in the security of the hospital.

I ring Dr Buckley. He tells me politely that I have to wait my turn and make an appointment through his secretary like everyone else. He used to drop everything for me. When I wrote to him, telling him I was going to give this diet a go, he was not encouraging and told me he had no faith in the treatment. But not only did he have no faith, he was put out and now he is just trying to make a point. This is the road I chose to take so I must suffer the consequences.

Elizabeth Beckett did say I would get worse before I felt better. She is caring, if a little busy. Maybe it is difficult to put me in touch with people? I must not be pathetic, nor give up at the first sign of trouble. I need to be patient and have more faith.

Sophie visits me in the evening. I have not been able to move from the sitting-room sofa all day. When she rang earlier to say she'd like to pop over, I couldn't even lift the phone to my ear, Mum had to rest it against me.

Jasmine, my new wire-haired dachshund, sits with her head burrowed underneath my arm. She has been attentive all day, sensing something is not right. I stroke her fondly.

'I can't bear to see you like this, are you sure this diet is the right thing?' Sophie asks with a familiar, anxious expression on her face.

'I don't know.' I need a good Samaritan to stop and pick me out of this ditch and on the right track again.

It's now the beginning of March and I am frightened. Mum's faith in the diet is fading, Dad's cynicism seems to be justified. My sense of isolation only increases further when Sophie leaves for Romania. She'll be away for three months .

'Don't go! Please stay. I can't face not having you around,' I sigh heavily. 'I'm selfish, aren't I?'

'I'll write,' she promises, putting her arms around me. 'You'll be OK and Seb will be back soon.'

'I've bought you a book to write your diary in. You can read it to me when you get back.'

'I got you these,' Sophie remembers, rummaging in her bag. She hands me some coffee beans, a large bar of dark chocolate and some grapefruit bubblebath.

'Soph, you know I love these things but I can't have them.'

She blushes. 'How much longer are you going to carry on with this diet thing?'

I can feel the tears choking my throat.

'Write to me, Ali, I'll want to know how you are.'

We go out to her car and I sit in the front seat. 'I wish I could come with you,' I say. All I can think of is the song, 'Ten green bottles hanging on the wall, and if one green bottle should accidentally fall, there'll be nine . . .' I feel like the bottle which is always on the shelf, watching all the others fall to a more exciting place. 'You must go, I'm going to start crying . . . I'm pathetic.' I give Sophie a big hug. Tears are in her eyes. 'Go . . . GO!' I smile. I cannot stand it, I am going to cry as well. I watch her move off into the distance and slowly turn back towards the house, feeling far from a whole person.

The next morning I'm at work, staring into my nettle tea. Have I been lulled into a false sense of security? Why haven't the diet, the fungi tea, the Epsom Salts, the oils helped me at all? I feel angry and let down. I have followed it religiously and it's failed. I walk boldly into the kitchen and pour the nettle tea down the sink, finally taking the decision to give up. I make myself a cup of filter coffee and enjoy every mouthful. On the way home I stop off at the BP service station and buy a king-size Mars bar and before paying for it I find that I've ripped off the wrapper, mouth watering at the sight of rippled chocolate coating gooey nougat and caramel.

Medical Update:
Dr Buckley has upped the dose of methotrexate which I continue to take with sulphasalazine.

27

'It's like the colour of your eyes'

I stare at the questions. *Are you able to run errands and shop?* I cannot tick 'without ANY difficulty' any more. I have moved on to the next two lines, which I didn't even glance at before. Now I'm ticking 'with SOME difficulty' or 'with MUCH difficulty'.

I have given up my part-time work. I was missing too many days, and when I rang up to say that I could not make it into the office I felt like I was letting Richard down. 'But you're not, Alice, just tell him and he'll understand. Far better that than him thinking you're just slacking, taking days off for fun,' Mum argued with me. 'Richard won't treat you any differently.'

So, I told him. I knocked nervously on his door, hands trembling, and when he told me to sit down I felt sick with shame. 'I'm sorry I've been missing so many days,' I began.

'That's all right, just as long as we get a fill-in it's OK, don't worry about it,' he replied flippantly. I could tell he didn't really have time to talk, he was busy. I almost stood up and left, thinking that there was no need to tell him, but something told me to stay firmly put. He looked at me as if to say, 'So, anything else or can I get on?' I then told him in a haphazard way about the rheumatoid arthritis – I hate saying those ugly words, and he sat back, his face softened and he listened quietly. 'I'm so sorry,' he said simply, 'but I'm glad you told me.'

That evening, he rang from his car to find out if he had any messages. Afterwards, 'How are you feeling?' he asked tentatively. Mum was wrong about him treating me differently, things had changed already.

I left shortly after telling Richard, and the office gave me flowers and a leaving card signed by all of them. Although it was a relief not to have to struggle into work any more, I knew I would miss them.

Dr Buckley is still reading my medical notes. He looks up. 'Rheumatoid arthritis is a part of you. It's like the colour of your eyes, I can't change it. We just have to hope it will burn out or be kept at bay so that you can lead some kind of normal life,' Dr Buckley says.

'Don't lie!' I cry out angrily. 'I've seen my file. You're full of bullshit. I'll never play tennis again, that's obvious now.'

'Your case is very severe,' he admits, taken aback. 'But look, I can't predict anything. I can't look into a crystal ball and tell you what's going to happen. If I could I'd go to the races more often.'

His weak joke doesn't work this time.

'Don't go off and follow another crazy diet,' he pleads. 'Somewhere along the way we will find a drug that helps. These drugs can take a while before they take effect but don't lose heart. Something other than tennis is out there for you, it's around the corner. I promise.'

Nothing will replace my tennis. How can he say such a thing?

As Mum and I are driving home, we pass Bill, playing on our tennis court. We had a court built in our garden when we first moved here, five years ago. I hate looking at it. I can't bring myself to walk outside or go anywhere near it. Over the past few months Bill has been paying us by the hour to use our court for coaching and that money has been put towards the cost of my alternative treatment. Now, though, it's going to ARC, the research charity for arthritis.

Half of me thinks it's OK him using our court, as he has nowhere else to coach at the moment and Mum wants to help him out. 'After all, he was a wonderful coach to you, Alice,' she said, 'and I feel I'm doing something positive with the money.' But the stronger half of me hates Bill for being there.

I watch him play from the window and smile. It reminds me of when we used to play. I can feel his shots and his movements around the court. My mind can still play, but when I pick up my racket, my wrist collapses, I can't hold it. I want to break it. Why should anyone else use my racket? I don't want anyone using our court either, especially Bill, Mr Insensitive. He has made no effort to support me. Why should he be here? I see Bill looking up towards me and I duck. I don't want to see him.

This is torture. This is my hell. I have to leave home, I am going to apply for a place at Bristol University. Sophie is going there and all I know is that I have to get out of here.

28

Seb

After seven months of travelling, Seb is back. I am seeing him tonight.

Part of me doesn't want to care. Over the last three months he has not written once. He is an insensitive bastard. However, when he rang at five o'clock this morning, telling me he had just landed, all the old feelings came flooding back. I think I do care, I want to see him.

I lie in the bath with a vodka and tonic to calm my nerves. Afterwards, I stand naked before my long mirror. Will Seb notice that my body has changed in the last seven months? The muscles which lie across the tops of my hands look as though they have been attacked ferociously with an ice-cream scoop. A few of my toes are bent like little claws. My swollen knees make my lower legs look like sticks and I have lost weight in my shoulders. I used to weigh nine and a half stone when I played tennis but now I weigh between seven and a half and eight. Will he love me any more? Maybe I want to tell Seb it's over because I am scared of intimacy, I am scared of sex.

I feel like an adulteress as I discard all traces of my life with RA. I throw out the cold hot-water bottle which sits at the bottom of my bed and I get rid of my hand splints, which are squashed under my pillow. My occupational therapist has given me weird contraptions and gadgets –

one of which is a long silver and grey stick with claw-like fingers that picks up things for you. I shove it into my wardrobe, together with the long white plastic shoehorn and the slimy green exercise putty for my hands. I hide my slippers, throw away empty packets of pills, pack the rest of my drugs into a make-up bag and put them in the cupboard in the bathroom. Then I lie down on my bed, feeling exhausted. My pillow inflates, making a gurgling noise and propelling me forward. Oops. I'd forgotten about that, it helps me sit up in the mornings. I pull out the controls and hide them under the bed. I lie down again and breathe deeply. Why am I bothering with all this? Seb may not even come back for the night.

'I'm sorry I didn't keep in touch as much as I should have done,' Seb apologizes over his pasta bowl.

We are eating out in an Italian restaurant. I purposely did not order spaghetti as I knew half of it would slurp on to my top. I'm eating lasagne with salad, although I can barely touch it. I'm picking at the salad like a nervous, twitchy little rabbit.

'No, no, it's OK,' I find myself saying, when I had planned to give him a hard time. I have butterflies in my stomach. I want to be in bed with him right now. Alice! I pinch myself under the table. Stop being so easy. He has not been Mr Wonderful. He must earn you again.

'I've missed you,' he says tentatively.

I've missed you too, take me now, I want to shout. I have to pinch myself again. I must play hard to get.

There's silence. 'I know I haven't been supportive.' Another long silence and he quickly changes the subject. 'What have you been up to?'

My face freezes like ice. I do not want to get into what

I've been doing. Nervously I pull the sleeves of my black ribbed cardigan down over my hands so that only my long fingers and nails show. Yet another awkward pause. 'I've been missing you,' I confess finally.

He smiles his wide smile and leans across the table, kissing me on the lips. I don't pull away and my heart jumps at his touch.

As the tension eases, Seb begins to talk about his travelling experiences. As he's talking, I am wondering what's going to happen this evening. Where do we go from here? I'd rather he shut up. I don't want to hear about bungee jumping, white-water rafting, hitch-hiking, or his immediate plans to travel around Europe – it only fills me with longing and envy. I just want him to take me home and rip my clothes off. I've missed sex. The anticipation alone makes me feel excited.

But at the same time, I'm terrified. I can't fling my clothes off any more. I've squeezed my feet into cowboy boots which are impossible to get off and I know I'll have to use the boot jack. I am not wearing the right clothes at all, why didn't I think this through? And will sex hurt now? Seb's six foot two and a rugby player. I'll be like one of those squashed-fly biscuits after he's through with me.

Seb's talking about barbecues, drinking sessions and camping on the beach with a group of backpackers he met along the way. I don't dare ask if he met anyone. If he says he has met someone and it's serious, than I have too. OK, my new man is . . .

'Alice, hey, calling Alice . . .' Seb's waving his hand in front of my face. 'Well, what do you think then?'

'Um, sorry, didn't catch the last bit.'

'About us? You're miles away, I thought you'd be happy to see me,' he says dejectedly.

I look at his gorgeously tanned face and white blond hair. He looks like Brad from *Neighbours*. Oh shit, my life is sad, I think, remembering how I watched *Neighbours* twice in one day the other week. What the hell. I grab Seb's hand. 'I am happy to see you. Come on, we need to make up for lost time. Let's go home.'

We giggle as we climb the stairs. 'Ssh, Seb, we'll wake Mum and Dad.' Seb picks me up and throws me on to the bed like in the movies. Only it hurts. He yanks my cowboy boots off, in the process pushing my feet down and bending my toes. I want to scream but instead I'm holding the pain inside. He pulls off my red T-shirt, thank God I'm wearing my black Wonderbra. Seb twists me round, quickly undoing my belt.

'Turn out the lights,' I say.

'No, I want to see you properly. I haven't seen you for a whole seven months.'

I take a deep breath. Will he still think I've got a good body? He's undoing my bra and kissing the back of my neck, my ears.

'You're thinner,' he says, his arms around my waist. 'Just as long as you don't lose weight here,' he says, kissing my breasts before moving lower and lower . . .

'It's more exciting in the dark,' I say, reaching to turn off the lights. I can't let him see me naked, he'll notice my swollen knee, and I don't want this to stop . . .

'Come back here,' he says. I hold the pain in again as he tugs at my hands. 'I've missed you so much,' he says, as he pulls me down into his arms.

My body is crying for sleep, every inch feels as if it has been pushed up against a wall and punched relentlessly. My legs shake as I walk to the bathroom and swallow two painkillers. I pray Seb won't wake up as I walk slowly back to the bed. He must not see the other half of me – a half which I feel is shameful, not good enough and unattractive.

Light creeps through the curtains. Seb moves restlessly on to his other side. I nestle next to him and look at his body. I would love to jump into it. Be tall, strong and fit. He turns from one broad tanned shoulder to the other. It is a wonderful release to have someone else to think about, and it was fantastic to have sex again. I loved it. I feel a great sense of relief too, I can still manage it! I can still just about flex my cranky body into different positions. I feel normal. NORMAL. One night with Seb has given me back the confidence I have lost over the last year. I wrap my arm around his waist, his hand opens to take mine, our soft fingers intertwining like a perfect puzzle. He says sleepily he loves me. My eyes close, shutting out the burning discomfort all over my body. I feel gloriously happy; being with him takes me back to the time when we first went out. He makes me feel like the girl I was without the RA.

Medical Update:
My ESR – Erythrocyte Sedimentation Rate, which signifies how active the disease and inflammation is, is 129. My doctor is worried. He tells me that anything over 100 is extraordinarily severe. I am also anaemic. A steroid drip and blood transfusion are both needed. Reassessing treatment with new doctor: replacing sulphasalazine with Drug Number 6, penicillamine. Replaced indomethacin with Drug Number 7, Voltarol. Persevering with the higher dose of methotrexate.

29

'Why ME?'

May 1993. I have got a place at Bristol University! Hurray. Seb has disappeared again and is now in France. I have just started seeing a genius doctor, Dr Fischer, in a hospital outside Bristol. My parents and I decided it was time to seek a second opinion and I'll need a doctor near the university. Dr Fischer wants me admitted into hospital for six weeks. I trust him and I am willing to give this a try. If he can't make me better, no one can. This is the beginning of a new life.

The new hospital has an unusual set-up. You do not fester in bed all day in your pyjamas, eating grapes and watching chat shows and soap operas. You are allowed to go out, provided you tell a nurse. There is a snack bar a few painful footsteps away which is becoming my second home. The waiter gently takes off my coat and helps me sit down, bringing me a cappuccino with extra grated chocolate and a few biscuits. You are also allowed to go home at the weekends.

At the beginning of my second week, I feel as if I am a weekly boarder at a school for sick people.

I spot the duty nurse, Gloria, who is looking after me. She is a wonderful character – a big black lady with huge waggling hips and a smile that could cheer the saddest of souls. 'How you doing, Alice?' she booms. 'Nice to have you back. What you been up to?'

'Nothing much,' I smile.

'Nothing! That sounds boring,' she says laughing, her bottom wiggling up and down.

'I went to a ballet but the best part was a Magnum ice-cream in the interval.'

'Oh, All-yce,' she says in a shrill tone, 'my husband says I should go on a diet, he thinks I'm too fat.'

She holds her tummy in for a second before exploding into giggles.

I am told a new turnover of people will be in the ward for my second week – a group of ankylosing spondylitis patients. Ankylosing spondylitis is a form of arthritis that affects the spine. They're arriving at teatime but I do not get a chance to see them as I have to go down to the hydrotherapy pool.

I am kicking my legs furiously up and down in flippers in the warm water. Mentally I am trying to kick and shake the RA out of my body.

As I am being wheeled back into the ward I notice one of the new ladies staring at me. She is young and pretty, with brown curly hair falling over her face. I sit down on my bed and look over at her again.

'Come and talk to me, darling, I'm Sally. What is it you have, love?'

'Rheumatoid arthritis,' I say, walking over to her bed.

'I thought it might be. I can see it in your face and your eyes. It's a look I used to have.' She pauses and blows her nose. I can see tears. 'I was diagnosed with that when I was young too, I was thirteen. It was awful, I could never play games at school and everyone in my class used to laugh and tease me. At night I shared a bed with my sister and she would rub my feet and legs up and down because I was in such pain. I was only taking aspirin but the drugs are more advanced now, research has moved forward.'

'I hope they find a cure quickly.'

She nods in sympathy. 'Don't give up. They will find something.'

I tell her about my tennis. She tells me how she used to love gymnastics but had to give it up. For the first time I realize that there are other people in the same boat. Others not sailing exactly where they would have liked. Life is not always mapped out according to your dreams but we are passengers who can help each other. She is young too, in her early thirties, and has suffered for most of her childhood and adult life. This is great, I am not the only *young* person putting up with this illness. For the first time I do not feel so alone.

I can't look as the thick needle is injected into my arm. It is in preparation for a blood transfusion. I have had this before: a bag of blood is pumped into me at a very slow rate, it takes four hours per bag, and I need four bags. Wherever I go, I have to take my drip with me. It's becoming a friend.

Fourth bag. My face looks alarmingly red and I feel drunk. The nurse tells me I must get into bed and rest. Bed?! I feel wide awake, hyperactive. Whose wonderful blood am I having? Maybe Steffi Graf's or Linford Christie's, or better still, Claudia Schiffer's. While you're at it, give me a body like hers too. It's an extraordinary feeling knowing that my system is being flushed out and new blood is being pumped into me. Helen wrote to me recently saying, 'It's lucky your character is not contained in your blood otherwise you would be a complete schizo-phrenic!'

I never gave blood when I was well but now I can see how important it is. I'm going to tell Andrew and Helen, and my friends, to give blood immediately.

The following morning I'm due for a steroid drip, and am looking forward to it immensely as I know it will help the pain. My disease LOVES steroids. It has a huge appetite for them.

Overnight the steroids work their magic. I feel like a new person. I don't feel as if I was run down by a double-decker bus in the night. This morning I threw the bedcovers off and showered straight away, I didn't want to stay in bed. My body feels so light and walking is much easier. I can see my ankles rather than a mound of fluid like an orange attached to my foot. Where does the fluid go?

Friends and family send cards. Helen sends me a card every day, Monet's *Sunrise* was one of them because she knows it's my favourite, and she tells me she does not want me looking unpopular in the ward. Rebecca writes from Australia, where she has been snorkelling along the Barrier Reef. Tom writes a letter from his community in St David's, Wales, asking how my legs are and telling me he's been to a Bible reading class and that he cooked sausages for supper. I think he is happy. Andrew sends a card from London, where he works. I can never read his writing – it looks like an inky spider has crawled across the page. Granny sends flowery cards, picked out for her by the lady who owns her local post office. There's something incredibly touching about her messages, written in wobbly handwriting, sending her fondest love and prayers.

Seb has not written for a while. His last letter was distanced. Right at the end he wrote, 'Hope you are well,' as if he were a stranger. His words felt empty. Well, at least he has not lost touch completely, I think. When I look at some of the patients in their beds, they have no cards or flowers. Does anyone care about them? It makes me feel sad.

Sophie is still in Romania. Late one night I turn on my light and write her a ten-page letter (unfortunately she never receives it because the post out there is so bad). I miss her.

The beginning of week four. The steroid pulse is already beginning to wear off. I feel like a caged animal. I ask Mum to take me shopping, retail therapy is needed desperately. Mum takes me out in the wheelchair, she tells me it will be less tiring for me. I don't mind, as I'm unlikely to bump into anybody I know. Just getting out of the hospital makes me feel better, seeing the outside world and feeling that I am part of it again. We have lunch in a French café and then head for Jigsaw, Ghost and Warehouse, Mum bumping me up and down on the grey pavements. In Jigsaw I buy a long black skirt, a white top and a dark red jumper. It is Helen's birthday soon and she is having a party at home. I should be out of hospital for good by then. The party will be fun and I will wear one of the tops then, I decide happily.

Helen and a couple of her girlfriends are helping with the cooking. I am sitting with them in the kitchen, drinking coffee. We are talking about boys and how hopeless they are. Mum is exhausted and eventually we persuade her to have a rest with a book and hot-water bottle in bed. Hospitals have a really draining effect.

Kitty is Helen's flatmate. She's gorgeous and great fun. She makes profiteroles that do not rise and they look more like squashed pancakes sandwiched together with cream.

I go upstairs to get changed. I put on my new long black skirt which flows down to my ankles. It covers up the lumps and bumps and no one will be able to see my bruised legs and fat knees. My lovely lime green short dress has been pushed to the back of my wardrobe, and sits there collecting dust. I go downstairs. I am looking forward to the party.

Everyone starts arriving at seven o'clock. It is a sit-down supper. Helen and I planned the seating together, putting pictures of famous people above the names. I am Kate Moss. Helen's Michelle Pfeiffer, of course, and Kitty's Delia Smith. Hosting parties does have its advantages.

The supper is delicious and I am enjoying myself. Helen's friends ask how I am in a kind and genuine way; Kitty's profiteroles travel round the table again and again as Helen whispers, 'Don't take one, pass them on.'

However, as the evening progresses, I begin to feel exhausted and snippets of conversation start to pass me by.

'I went skiing in Val d'Isère, it was wonderful,' says one.

'Congratulations about the engagement, by the way,' says another.

'How's the job going?'

'Did I tell you I got on to *Blind Date*, it's going to be such a laugh. I met some lovely people at the interviews too. I'll be on TV soon, can you believe it?!'

Well, that does it. Why have they all got such interesting, fun lives? I am watching everyone enviously. Why not one of them, why me? What do I have to smile about? Nothing. Who can I talk about? Fat nurses and Doctor Fischer, whom I hardly see anyway.

'Did you hear that, Alice? Elaine's getting married in a couple of months.' I fake a smile and down a whole glass of wine in one go.

The party is getting louder and louder. One of the girls starts to strip and dance around the table, waving her bra in the air. Helen decides to join in. Stereo MC is on full blast, the table is cleared and everyone is dancing. I try to dance but I hear my right hip crunch. In fear, I put my hand over it and collapse back down on to my chair.

While no one is looking, I lift my skirt. My knee has doubled in size. Slowly I walk to the bathroom, hearing my hip crunch again. The noise terrifies me. What is happening to my body? It is falling apart like crumbly pastry. I swallow two painkillers and stare at my reflection. My face is flushed from the alcohol and it's fat from the steroid. I look like a drunk chipmunk. Purple shadows hang like half-moons under my blue eyes. I thought I looked pretty tonight, but the only thing I like is my long, thick hair. I tie it back and a clump falls into my hand. Gasping with shock, I touch my hair again and another clump comes loose. It's the poisonous drugs I'm on, I think angrily as I lock the door, my fingers trembling. I sit on the loo, crying. I can't go back out and I don't want to join the party. I can hear them all laughing, dancing. I envy their quick steps. I envy their lives.

Eventually I slip out of the bathroom and go upstairs to bed. No one will notice I've gone, they're having too much fun. I undress and throw myself into bed. I can't be bothered to brush my teeth, I don't care any more, I just want to be unconscious.

The following day the sun is shining, everyone is hungover and feeling sorry for themselves. The party went on all night. A pub lunch by the river is suggested but I do not go, choosing instead to stay with Mum.

'Why didn't you go, love? You would have enjoyed it,' she says, kneading dough for some scones for tea. Mum always seems to be making scones – I call it her 'nervous disease'.

'Why should I go? I've got nothing to contribute, they don't want me there,' I spit angrily, ripping a piece of scrap paper to shreds.

'You know that's not true,' Mum disagrees firmly. 'Well, be useful and help me cut some more scones.'

'I hate myself, I hate my life. I'm always in bloody hospital. I'm no better. Why, why me? Why, Mum?' I explode. 'It's not fair, I hate it, hate it, hate it.' Her rolling-pin flattens the pastry with extra force.

Helen's party returns after lunch on great form. They decide to have a game of tennis to blow the cobwebs away, get rid of the hangovers and run off the big Sunday roast. Are they doing it on purpose? Do they know how I feel? I am watching miss-hits and clumsy shots going way out. No one can play like I used to – so why me? Why can't I play any more? Why am I the one watching? I begin to wish passionately that I had never played. I can't bear the sense of loss which haunts me each day, eating into me.

One of them suddenly shouts, 'Alice, I could do with some tips from a pro,' thinking that will make me feel better. It makes me feel worse. I walk off, pretending I haven't heard. All I can think about is how I ought to be in America playing tennis, playing in international tournaments. I ought to be fit and healthy. I ought to be the one running around.

When Helen's friends have left, I walk down to the tennis court with my old Wilson racket and I stand on the baseline. 'I can still play,' I think to myself. I hold the ball in front of me and hit it. My wrist collapses. The ball does not even reach the net. I try harder, only inflicting more pain. I can't believe this is me.

I walk back up to the house, choked with anger and tears. I go inside and turn on the television. It's bloody tennis, Wimbledon. My contemporaries are playing. Shirli-Ann Siddall, the girl I played at the Nationals in Wimbledon, nearly beat Jennifer Capriati. Karen Cross, with whom I used to bed and breakfast during the nationals, is playing at Wimbledon for the first time. We used to have close matches. I should be there. I didn't realize what I had, how lucky I was to be able to play. And now it's gone. Gone for ever. Steffi wins a tight match, she's rushing to the net, a few tears collecting in her eyes. I miss winning, I miss that sense of triumph and achievement. I can't watch it. I slam the controls down.

Feeling like an old woman, I walk upstairs to my bedroom, wishing I could lock myself in for ever. I cry solidly for an hour and hurt my hand hitting my pillow. I don't even have the strength to throw things around, for fuck's sake. Instead I scream. No one can hear me, they are all outside.

Suddenly Dad comes in. 'Alice.' I don't think he knows what else to say. He sits next to me on the bed. I try and hurl another pillow on to the floor, screaming, sobbing, losing my breath I am crying so much. 'Let it all out, let it all out,' he says, stroking my back.

'My life's worth nothing. I can't play tennis. I can't dance, I can't run around, I can't go skiing, I can't get a job like all of them. I can't go on *Blind Date*. Imagine Cilla saying, "Alice you're going on a rock–climbing holiday, or white-water rafting, or skiing in the Alps." The oldies on that show can do more than me.' I begin to choke on my words. Finally, 'I can't do anything, Dad.'

I look at the bottle of pills on my bedside table. Why aren't they helping me? I pick the bottle up and throw it across the room. The bottle smashes against the wall, the pills hit the floor. 'Why aren't you doing anything?' I scream. 'Why is everyone living except me? I'm nineteen!'

Dad hangs his head and breathes deeply. He is holding his hands together in prayer.

'Your prayers do nothing! Don't bother. I have no faith,' I say vehemently. 'I don't know how you can still believe either. He's a cruel God. An evil God. You're fooling yourself.'

'Ssh, ssh,' Dad soothes, understanding the sting to my words. 'This weekend's been hard for you. But you're going to get better my darling, darling girl. I will make sure of that. You will manage at Bristol. I love you so much, you know that, don't you?'

'Why me, Dad? Why ME? I've never done anything wrong. Tom's right. It's the devil playing games. We are toys he can have fun with.'

Dad sighs. 'God is not sitting on his throne handing out punishments to the baddies. It does not work like that.'

'So where is he? On holiday?'

'Believe me,' he replies sharply, 'there are times when

I scream at him, I shout, "Why aren't my prayers working? Why doesn't the medication help? Why should Alice have to suffer like this?" But,' he says more calmly, 'I think he is still suffering in people and situations. I think he will for as long as this world exists.'

'I still don't think I believe that,' I say, my tears beginning to dry.

'I was reading a story about some Jewish children who had been hanged during the Holocaust. Someone who saw them turned round to his companion, breaking down, crying, 'Where is God? Why doesn't he stop it?' His friend replied, 'God is hanging right next to them.'

After a long pause. 'I'll never know the answer to why me, will I?'

'Not a minute goes by when I don't wish it was me, not you,' Dad says softly, a stream of silent tears flowing from his eyes. 'I'll never know the answer to, "Why not an old grey-haired man like me who's had half his life?"'

'I'm glad it's not you, Dad,' I say, coughing weakly.

'Why not an old man like me?' Dad repeats, cradling me in his protective arms.

30

Illness Shame

'Will I be able to go to Bristol?' I ask Dr Fischer. 'I mean, what happens if I have a dreadful flare-up?'

'You will manage,' he says resignedly. He leans back in his chair and crosses his short stumpy legs. 'You are in the best care here. I don't think you have anything to worry about, the higher dose of methotrexate ought to control your arthritis, it's a wonderful drug, very successful in America.'

'I don't like him,' Mum says after the appointment. 'You ask him what you think is a perfectly reasonable question and he makes you feel like a squashed grasshopper.'

'He talks like a King,' I say, smiling. 'Let's call him the Fischer King. Well, if the King says I'll be OK, I'll be OK.'

I am in my halls of residence, hiding in my dingy cardboard box of a room. Rebecca travelled up from home with me, as she too is at Bristol. We were both apprehensive and made a pact that we would keep in touch even though our halls are miles apart. It is strange the way we always end up together. From childhood we have shared in each other's lives and her family are like my second family.

I look at the mouldy brown curtains, the empty

wardrobe, the magnolia walls. I look at all the luggage waiting to be unpacked.

Mum begins to hang my clothes in the wardrobe. I wish she'd go, I hate goodbyes. I tell her to stop, that I can manage. I ask Mum and Dad to go, we hug and I know Mum is crying when her back is turned.

They've gone. Immediately I dig out my photographs in frames and start hanging them up. I have one of Helen, Mum, Dad, Tom and Andrew, one of Sophie and one of Seb and me taken after our A level results. I saw Seb just before leaving for Bristol and we decided it was over — we have both moved on. It was sad saying goodbye and I miss having a boyfriend. My insecurities make me question whether things would have been different had I not had RA, but we never spoke about it. Our relationship changed irrevocably when he went away for the second time.

I hold the photograph of my parents hugging on the day of their twenty-fifth wedding anniversary. Dad's cheeks look pink from drink, his eyes are laughing. It was a happy time, I was well. I feel a lump in my throat.

I can hear the hustle and bustle outside. I don't want to leave my room yet. I want to hide in here for ever and feel scared of the outside world. How am I going to cope at Bristol if I can't talk to people? How am I going to mix with people my age?

Suddenly Sophie bursts in and opens the curtains, 'Al, you haven't unpacked yet, look, we've got the best views. Are you all right?'

'Yes, fine.'

'Look, I'm here for you and if you're feeling bad I'll help,' she reassures me. Sophie wrote a letter to the warden in the summer, asking whether she could be near

me to give support and help. 'And Marcus is here.'
Marcus is a great friend from home, Sophie went out
with his twin brother.

'I know, I'm being stupid. Listen, I don't want anyone
to know about my RA. I'll tell people when I'm ready.
Can you imagine starting conversations by saying, "Hey,
I have rheumatoid arthritis." No one will want to know.'
Pause. 'I just don't want people to know.'

'I won't say anything if you don't want me to, although
I think you should.'

I look at her with pleading eyes. 'You won't tell anyone yet, will you?'

'Come on, let's go to the bar. We both need a drink.'

The bar is crowded. Everyone is shouting to be heard
over the music. Freedom and excitement at being away
from home fill the air. Boys are playing pool, groups of
people are talking and a few others are drunk already and
dancing. A boy with brown hair, tall and thin and dressed
in a blue checked shirt and jeans, comes up to us. His
shoes make a loud clicking noise on the floorboards. He
is not shy at all, immediately chatting us up, asking if we
want another drink and a game of pool. 'By the way, my
name's Matthew, but you can call me Matt,' he adds,
smiling at me as if this were a huge compliment. We go
over to the pool table.

I can hear voices from all directions. I switch off.

'I'm on A floor, come up later, we're having a gin and
tonic party,' says one.

'Look at that girl in the leather jeans over there.
Phwoar!'

'What course are you doing?' another asks.

'Whose round is it?'

'See my mate over there, he's brilliant at tennis, he plays for Gibraltar. Beats the shit out of me.'

'Do you like sport?' Matthew asks, poking me on the shoulder. 'How about a game of doubles?' He is looking at me. The question is directed at ME.

Later, trying to sleep, my reply haunts me. 'I'm not really interested in sport, I'm really quite lazy, I'm not that good at tennis.' I reach over to get the picture Bill took of me in Miami after I had won the tournament. It is in one of my favourite silver photograph frames. I hold it close to me. My tennis days now seem little more than a dream. I want my old life back, I want to play like I used to, I can't believe I'll never play again. I turn out the light and hug the photograph to my chest. 'Dear God, give me my life back, give me my life back,' I pray. I don't want to let the frame go. The following morning I wake up disorientated, the photo frame has fallen to the floor. After a few moments I remember where I am and stay in bed for another hour.

The Halls of Residence Committee has organized barn dances, discos, sporting events, balls with gladiators and bouncy castles, three-legged pub crawls. It's very nice of them, but each one demands the use of arms and LEGS. There should be a separate list for cripples like me.

Freshers' Week, Tuesday. Representatives from various societies congregate in the Student Union touting for our membership. Sophie wants to join the netball team, so we battle up some stairs to enter the sports section where voices ring out.

'Come and join the skiing society – we're going to Meribel this Christmas.'

'Any girls interested in rugby?'

'Sign up for tennis, we need a good team this year.'

I feel sick. Everything and everyone is turning on me. I have a desperate urge to kick the tables over, scream and shout. What *am* I doing here?

By the end of the week my feet feel as if they have been fighting – under protest – in a major war. I take my socks off, the toes are battered soldiers. They are squashed up and blistered. Two of my toes are in love – they practically lie on top of each other. Another toe is so bent it has rubbed against my shoe and is now red and raw. The edge of the sock leaves an indent. I can press the fluid in my ankles and feet, it feels squishy. Then the fluid rises again like dough and I make patterns with it. I look at my feet in disgust. They are ugly, I'm becoming flat-footed and all the toes are dislocated.

I know more or less why this is happening. The muscles, tendons and ligaments around the bones help the foot to remain supple and are also responsible for the movement of the toes. In a normal foot, the tendons pull in a straight line. With swollen joints in the feet, the tendons are pushed to one side, causing the muscles to move sideways and leading to deformity of the toes. What kind of monster does this to your body?

I feel like Cinderella's ugly sister as I try to squash my feet into trainers. Walking to the phone box, one hundred feet down the corridor, feels like walking barefoot across a beach, shells and sharp pebbles digging in with every step. I stand still and the pain lingers, meanders around my feet and ankles, travels up to my knees and hips. It waits for the next move, the next shot. At the end of my journey, I lean against the wall, out of breath, and dial Helen's number. I scream inside as I listen to the engaged tone. Get off the phone, Helen, I panic, stabbing at the numbers desperately. I can't go away and come back again. I dial for the fifth time.

'Hi, are you having a fantastic time?' she asks.

'No!' I screech immediately, before lowering my voice. 'Oh Helen, it's been awful, nothing like I imagined.' I tell her about the week.

'Go and see Dr Fischer. You can't go on like this. Don't put a brave face on it all the time, it won't help in the long run.'

'Well, your treatment should be kicking in by now,' Dr Fischer says, flicking through the pages of my medical notes with his well-manicured nails. 'There's nothing else I can do,' he says coolly.

'Nothing?' I ask incredulously. I notice the hairs protruding from his nostrils. 'My lectures start at nine next week. How am I going to get to them? I only just managed to keep this three o'clock appointment.'

'Well, I suggest you go to bed earlier and get up earlier.' He closes his file, as if to say, 'Thank you, that will be all.'

I want to shake him, hit him, pull out his perfect curly blond hair at the roots, kick him into action. But he has that look about him which suggests there is a bad smell in the room. He makes me feel unworthy of breathing the same air as him.

'But can't he look at your medication again?' Sophie asks as we drive back to Bristol. 'Can't he try something else, give you stronger painkillers, anything?' She is growing more irritated with each passing minute.

'I wish I liked him more, Soph,' I say, sighing deeply. 'I know he's a good doctor, he's like a bible of medical knowledge, but we can't communicate. I can't talk to him. It's useless and I don't know what to do. Why doesn't Dr Buckley have a twin doctor who lives in Bristol? '

'So inconvenient of him!' Sophie smiles, as we see the lights of Clifton ahead.

Second week, the beginning of lectures. The lecture halls are half a mile away, I have managed to pick the hilliest university city. Travelling from A to B is not one of my strong points, so how am I going to get there? My options are limited:

1 Get a taxi. However, £6.50 × 365 = £2,372. 50.
2 Buy some roller blades – but if I fell I don't think I could get up again.
3 Ask a genius to make me a wooden petticoat on wheels (a clever suggestion made by my uncle Peregrine) so I can roll down the hills.
4 Hitch-hike.
5 Walk.
6 Don't bother.

Option 6 is the most tempting but I think it has to be option 5. I'll get up at five in the morning, wolf down a few doughnuts, pack my bag and take a torch with me. I can hobble as slowly as I like because no one will be watching and, when I arrive at nine, I can pretend to have 'legged' it like everyone else because of a late night and hangover.

Oops, I overslept on the first day of my great plan and simply jumped into a taxi instead.

'Why are you getting a taxi to lectures?' one of the boys asks me that morning. 'It's not far!'

'Because I'm rich and spoilt,' I say.

He looks at me blankly.

'Don't tell me you walk?' I don't think he can believe his ears. This could be fun!

Later in the day, I am crawling like a snail from lectures to the library.

'You're limping,' observes someone behind me.

I turn round, my heart thumping. It's Matthew. He's been running and his forehead is shiny. He puts his hand through sweaty hair. 'Are you OK? Here, let me take your books. Why are you limping?' he asks, still jogging up and down. His energy makes me feel quite tired.

'I've got these great new shoes but they give me really bad blisters.'

'What?! They don't look new,' Matthew says, looking at my tatty leather loafers.

'They are new! Cost me two hundred pounds,' I say, pretending to be offended.

His face drops. 'You shouldn't walk in them if they hurt.'

'I'm vain, I don't mind the pain.'

I can hardly move. I feel like the creaky tin man in *The Wizard of Oz*, badly in need of oiling. The rats are already in my body, beating down on my joints with hot hammers, attacking them relentlessly, biting into them. It's eight o'clock in the morning and my lecture starts at ten. I circle my neck round and round, I shrug my shoulders and stretch my legs, hearing the knees snap like wafers. I stand up. My hip sounds like crackling, splintered wood, the cartilage which protects the joint has been eroded and the bones are grating against each other because they have no cushioning. I limp to my door and open it slightly to see if anyone is hanging around in the corridor. I am a detective on the look-out. All is clear, so I grab my grapefruit shower gel and towel and walk as quickly as I can to the shower room.

I step into the shower and try to turn the switch on. Water begins to flow eventually, but it's boiling, scalding, and I can't stay under it although I need to rinse the soap off. I can't change the temperature because the switch is too stiff. I can't even turn it off. There's steam everywhere. I step out, clutching my towel around me, and begin to walk back to my room, flustered and soapy. I can hear someone and try to speed up. I dart into my room, but, no, I'm in the linen cupboard. I come out, Matthew sees me, and my towel slips off. Shit. I cover myself up quickly, hold my head down and go to my room, covered in soap and leaving soapy footprints in the corridor. Oh well, I like to make my mark. Glad to be of entertainment.

Matthew knocks on the door. 'Let me in, Alice.'

'Hang on a sec,' I say as casually as possible, while desperately trying to put my bra on.

He barges in. I now have my jumper stuck around my head. He pulls it down for me. 'What's going on? Are you OK or just really strange?'

'I'm fine but running really late. Sorry, Matt, I can't talk now.'

After the shower fiasco I have some breakfast. Every step I take is like walking on broken glass. I smile a ravishing smile at everyone and sit down with my Alpen. I then wait for everyone to leave before ringing for a taxi. I lie down on the back seat so that no one can see me and ask the taxi driver to drop me off just before we reach the lecture halls. I walk the last stretch, giving the impression I have walked the whole distance.

Five weeks into the term, I'm still pretending, lying and catching taxis. Not only am I an ill student, but also a very poor and unhappy one. Pain is a great separator, it forms a wall around you and I won't let anyone break down that wall. I want to believe I can cope and I don't want people treating me differently. I have to see Dr Fischer again about my hip. The noise and pain is running away with itself. I am scared of having another X-ray and witnessing further damage, but at the same time I know I ought to do something about it. He must help me, that's what doctors are for.

An appointment is made.

Naturally I bump into Matthew as Sophie and I are walking to our taxi, parked outside the front door of our halls of residence. 'Hi,' he smiles, 'where are you off to?'

I beam at him. 'Jigsaw.'

Matthew waves goodbye. 'Don't buy another pair of two-hundred-pound shoes,' he says. I'm sure he is suspicious.

'Hi, sit down,' Dr Fischer says, opening my file, which is now twice its original size. 'How are you feeling at the moment?'

'Terrible. I'm in pain virtually all the time.'

'Go into the changing-room. Let's have a look at these joints.' My heavy body peels itself off the chair. 'Would you mind taking your things with you? I don't want them on my desk,' he says, glancing at my bag.

'I'm sorry.' I pick up my bag and he sits back in his chair.

I hate showing him my body, it was never an issue with Dr Buckley. My hands hurt as I try to fold my clothes and put them on the chair to avoid any more clutter.

Dr Fischer comes in. He looks at my knees and ankles. 'Right, yes, there is swelling, but I don't think it's disastrous.'

'What about my hip?'

He pulls my knees up towards my chest to see what range of movement I have in the hips. 'Put your clothes back on and come into my room.'

'Is that it?' I gasp.

'Yes, I've seen all I need to see,' he says sharply.

I go into his office and try to explain again. 'Look,' I say, trying to keep calm, 'my hip's hurting. I don't want to be around other people because I am scared they will hear the clicking noise it makes. That's no way to lead a young life.'

He stares right through me.

'Is it going to get worse, is there anything that will help?' I persevere.

Finally all he can muster is, 'I'm cautious about doing anything with the hip, but I suppose I can increase your steroids.'

'That was quick,' Sophie says.

'Let's go,' I say firmly. Being near him makes me feel physically sick.

She gets up. 'What's wrong?'

'I should have said . . . oh, forget it, I can't talk to him, we have a chronic personality clash.'

'Do you want me to go in and see him?' Sophie cuts in. 'Maybe it will help if I . . .'

'No, I want to go.'

'Want one?' Sophie hands me a cigarette outside the hospital.

'Yes.' Thank God for cigarettes. Smoking may be bad for you, but it's not going to be the first thing to kill me.

When I ring home, the sound of Dad's familiar voice makes me cry. I wish I could shrink him and put him in my pocket. I miss his calm face, his guidance and wisdom. I need to share his unshakeable faith in the light at the end of the tunnel. I put the phone down and tears run down my cheeks. I am shaking. Just thinking about the day again makes me angry and upset. I open the door and Matthew is standing there, staring at me. 'Hey, what's wrong?' he asks. 'Come here.' He puts his arms around me. I do not care any more, I am not able to hide how miserable I am. 'Let's go and get a drink and you can tell me all about it,' he says softly.

Matthew pulls up a chair for me. 'Sit down. Here's your vodka and tonic.'

'Thanks, I'll be all right in a minute.'

'Don't lie any more,' he insists. 'Alice, I know what's wrong. Sophie told me, and don't get annoyed with her. She's really worried about you.'

'You know?' I say limply. 'Well, I can't pretend any more. I can't keep hiding in my room.'

'Why didn't you tell me? What did you think I'd do?'

'I don't know.' I realize suddenly that he's right. What could be the worst scenario of telling someone? They'd think I was a freak, run a mile, never talk to me again? Well, if they did, they wouldn't have been much of a friend in the first place.

'I can't believe it,' he says, when I tell him about my tennis. 'I sprained my ankle before the marathon and thought that was bad enough. I'm running this year though and I'm going to raise money for arthritis. I've never run for a friend before, it'll make me more motivated.' He rolls up his sleeves. 'Don't hide any more, you silly girl. People will want to help. I want to help.'

I look up. Why did I worry about telling people if this was the kind of response I was going to get? Walking back to halls, I let Matthew take my arm to support me and we carry on talking as if everything else is normal . . .

I am in a wheelchair, sitting in Dr Buckley's waiting-room. I am handed the familiar questionnaire.

'Are you able to walk outdoors on flat ground?'

I tick 'Unable to do'. A line I never dreamt I'd use.

My head feels like a lead ball, solid and heavy, pumped full with more steroids and drugs. I shake it around and I can hear the rattle of pills. My joints, like dominoes, are being attacked one by one – shoulders down to elbows down to hands, down to hips and knees, down to feet, down to toes. One push and they all follow. It's my hip now, but which joint will be next? What's going to happen when all the dominoes fall flat on the ground in a heap? Will I have to live for ever in this wheelchair? I never believed I would be so crippled with this disease.

My first term at Bristol is over. My body collapsed once I was at home, it was finally allowed to give in. I can no longer fight the pain, repress it, bottle it. The flare-ups are flowing one after the other. Mum struggled to get me into the car, every movement hurting. When we arrived at the hospital, she said she was going to get a wheelchair from one of the porters.

'No, I can walk, don't, Mum,' I pleaded.

'Don't be ridiculous, you're in agony. Wait there.' She walked off and I could see her asking one of the young porters for a chair. She was pointing at the car, at me. I felt embarrassed, but why should I feel so embarrassed? Somebody in a wheelchair is not an unfamiliar sight in hospital. Why struggle, you crazy, idiotic, dumb girl? But I felt ashamed at the thought of being pushed around. I was certain everyone's eyes would be on me, wondering what was wrong. I am not an invalid. Mum came towards me, the wheels rattling on the ground. I pleaded with her to take the wheelchair away. I don't want it.

'Let me walk, Mum. I can walk,' I said, trying to get up.

'It's too far to walk,' Mum repeated. 'Please, I'm too tired to argue.'

I looked at Mum. She is always there for me, her fighting spirit is enough to keep us both going. However, for the first time I saw lines of real fear and grief etched on her soft face. I plonked myself down. 'I'm sorry,' I said meekly.

'I know it's difficult,' she said, unlocking the brakes forcefully. 'I know it is.'

We trundled off to the Rheumatology Department, me biting my lip, head down, telling myself over and over, 'I'm too young, I'm too young, I shouldn't be here.' I know Mum was thinking to herself, 'I wish it was me, I wish it was me.'

Dr Buckley is looking at my recent hip X-ray. 'If I were you, I'd pin a surgeon up against the wall and tell him to operate straight away. You are young, but I don't think we should wait. Life's too short.' He holds the X-ray up against the light board again. 'The damage is dreadful. You need a total hip replacement, and soon.'

'How soon?'

'You've got to leave Bristol.'

31

Black

'It's the devil playing games,' Tom says. 'He plays games with our lives.'

Tom is at home for a short break. He is sitting on my bed reading horoscopes. 'Your financial matters need to be addressed and on the eighteenth you will meet . . .'

'Tom, it's a load of rubbish,' I sigh, hoping he'll shut up.

He tries to hug me. I scream. I don't want him to touch me. He withdraws, a few tears in his eyes. 'I can see the devil. He's sitting in his deepest, darkest den, in a really vile mood, making my sister sick.' His face clouds over. It is a look which tells me an outburst is on the way.

'Tom, go away,' I snap. I cannot cope with his black moods too.

It's the beginning of 1994. I'm at home. It's winter. It's cold, dark and depressing. I gave up my place at Bristol and I'm on a waiting list for a hip replacement operation.

Every day I hate waking up. I loathe my illness with a passion. I feel as if I'm in a dark dungeon, it's grimy, cobwebbed walls closing on me, shutting out any light.

It's ongoing torture. My useless body serves me only as a source of pain. Major surgery on the hip is only the first of many operations to come and I can't cope. My life would be a lot easier if I just ended it, at least then I would have enjoyed the majority of my time in this mysterious world. Why live a longer life clouded by illness and misery?

I curse myself for feeling like this, but however much I try to escape from the dungeon I slip back down the wall. Not even my parents or closest friends can throw down the rescuing rope, I know it has to come from within me. Yet I can't face it. I don't want to escape, entering a world where I still have RA. It's too bleak. If I can't be who I want to be, I don't want to be at all.

I know my parents are sick with worry. They feel helpless. On several occasions Mum mentions that I should see a counsellor but I get angry and refuse. I am so depressed, I do not want to help myself. My character has withered like a flower, the petals falling to the ground, one by one. A part of me has died.

I am having recurring nightmares. I am restless, tossing and turning in bed. One dream in particular haunts me like a ghost.

I am playing at Wimbledon, Centre Court, and Bill is at the net, taking it in turns to hit balls to each player. Charlotte is standing in front of me but it is my turn to hit the ball. I am not in the right clothes, I am wearing a tight, sequinned dress and stilettos. I try to move but I am stuck, my heels are dug into the ground. I lunge forward but my feet don't move. All eyes are on me.

'Move, Alice,' Bill is shouting. 'What's wrong with you?' he yells. Spectators are staring, laughing, pointing, jeering.

'Move, move, MOVE,' I shout in my sleep. I wake up, drenched in sweat.

★

I lie in bed concocting ways to kill myself.

I could take the car out, find a secluded place and swallow all of my pills in one go. It would all be over. Or, I could just crash into a fence, a hedge, hoping that it would finish me off for good because I don't want to survive with broken front teeth and a broken arm. I could try to hang myself but I don't think I'm strong enough to set it up. Things would be much easier if I only had a gun . . .

Alternatively, I could take all my pills tonight, go to bed and sleep for ever. 'Over, the end' – those words bring relief, they make me smile. I would rather be dead than live with rheumatoid arthritis. This is the answer, I have found my means of escape.

I perk up enormously knowing it will all be over soon. I sit up and begin to drink my tea, which is cold and stewed. Everyone's so nice about you when you die, I wonder what they'll say about me? They'll remember me as the wonderful tennis player, full of life and sparkle but cruelly stricken with RA at the beginning of a successful tennis career. If I carry on living, I'll only become 'Poor Arthritic Alice'. I do not know how Mum puts up with me as well as Tom, I hate being a burden. Well, soon she won't have to worry about me any more. It's best for both of us.

I get up, each step the equivalent to having a dagger thrust through the sole. As I am getting dressed, I notice that a nodule, a lump of swollen tissue under the skin, has settled on my left elbow. I also have one on my little finger. I look in the mirror – and I can only see fat knees, a puffy face and lumps on elbows. I cannot see *me* any more, just the arthritis. I lift up painful, locked shoulders and put on a sloppy red sweatshirt, exhausted by the effort of it all. I remember my plan and go downstairs humming a merry tune. 'Sorry about earlier, Mum,' I say breezily.

'How are you feeling?' she asks, putting down the phone.

'Just the same. My hip sounds like a clapped-out tractor.'

'Well, hopefully it's not long until the operation. It will make all the difference.' Silly old Mum. Does she not know it will all be over tomorrow?

I shrink like a snail withdrawing into its shell when the phone rings. I breathe a huge sigh of relief when I know the call is not for me. I don't want to speak to anyone.

The evening comes. I kiss Tom, Mum and Dad goodnight and give them an extra long hug. I get into my pyjamas, clean my teeth and open my box of painkillers. How many will I have to take? Twenty, fifty? I start popping them out of their silver packets. There are about forty in the box, hopefully that will be enough. What shall I swallow them with? I go downstairs and pinch a bottle of vodka.

I'm making pretty patterns on my bed with the white chalky pills – flowers, hexagons, faces. The moment has come. I hear the phone ring downstairs, 'Oh, Ma, it was my turn to call you,' Mum is saying to Granny. 'No, she's gone to bed. She's very low at the moment and we don't know what to do.'

Granny is a role-model of courage for our family. Mum draws strength from her support. What would Granny do if she were in my shoes? She would not give up, she would fight it. Granny went to Africa with nothing and, against huge odds, made a new life for herself.

I put my hands over my ears. I don't want to hear them talking, I don't want to feel guilty. Yet, if I go ahead with this, I am letting Granny, Mum, Dad, Helen, Sophie, all my friends and family down. Can I really bear not seeing them again?

I sit at the end of my bed, staring at the pretty array of pills and the untouched bottle of vodka. I should have done it by now. I have to go through with this. I pour the vodka into a glass and start to take the pills, holding a few up to my mouth, the sticky coatings of their man-made taste settling on my lips. I hold the glass of vodka in my other hand.

I see my reflection in the mirror. 'Go on, do it,' a voice is saying. 'What's the point of living? Swallow the lot, you can do it.'

I throw the pills down and they scatter across the floor. 'I can't do it,' I sob into my pillow. I feel a failure for not going ahead. A coward. Images of Mum and Dad's faces are haunting my mind. I can see their brave smiles, hear Mum's infectious laugh, feel their tears. I don't want to be thinking rationally, I want to be insane and not consider the repercussions. This is supposed to be about me, I think desperately, but I can't help thinking what it would do to my parents. It would kill them, not me.

I can't do it.

When I wake up the following morning, my pills are still scattered on the floor like seeds. I didn't move them, I wanted Mum to see them. At last she comes into my bedroom.

'Why are your pills out?' she asks. I do not know what to say. I'm angry at myself for not going through with it. 'I should have swallowed them,' I say miserably.

Mum is furious. 'Alice, you have two choices. You

can either give up and end your life . . . or you can live. I can see why you are depressed and low, anyone would be, but you cannot go on like this. I won't have it. I have organized for someone to come and see you, I can't force you to see her and at the end of the day it is up to you, but you know how I feel.' She storms out of the room.

'Who is she?' I call after her. 'Mum, come back, please. Who is she?'

Mum stands at my door, 'Her name's Jenny.'

32

Jenny

Not only have I got RA, I'm now a nutcase seeing a shrink.

Mum pushes me outside in my wheelchair, she says the fresh air will do me good. I am waiting for this Jenny person to come and see me and I am actually looking forward to seeing her, although naturally I remain indifferent on the outside. No way am I going to tell Mum this might be a good idea, that she might have been right all along. I wonder what Jenny looks like, what she is going to say to me. What am I going to say to her? I have never done anything like this before. I hope I will like her and that she will like me.

'I think she's here,' Mum calls. 'I'll get another chair, you can stay outside.'

'Great,' I shrug, avoiding eye contact with Mum.

Jenny comes through the gate. She is tall, a willowy figure with light blonde hair. Mum introduces herself. 'And here's Alice. Alice, this is Jenny. Can I get you anything?'

'A glass of water would be lovely,' Jenny replies. She has a kind face. 'Hello,' she says. I decide that she is also a little nervous.

'Hi,' I smile. There is an awkward pause. Do I say anything or do I wait for her to ask me something?

She breaks the silence, 'I'm so sorry to hear that you

were diagnosed with rheumatoid arthritis. I know it is very painful.'

'It is. I never knew pain like this existed.'

'Would you like to tell me about it?'

'Where do I start?' I ask, breathing deeply and drinking my water nervously. Jenny waits for me to go on. 'I can't believe I have it, I'm too young. I miss my tennis. I was a National player.'

'You obviously had a great gift and you feel it was taken away from you.'

'Yes, I feel punished. I don't deserve to have this. I don't think I'd even inflict it on my worst enemy. Tom says Saddam Hussein ought to have it. Why did it happen? That's what really gets me.'

'I don't know, it's unfair. Sometimes things don't make sense.'

'I didn't have an accident, no virus triggering it off, I wasn't stressed out. I was excited about the future and America. Why, *why* did it happen?' I say, a lump in my throat. 'Now I . . .' I stop in my tracks. I feel ashamed about last night, I feel ashamed that I wanted to take my life.

'Now what?'

'I don't want to carry on, I don't want a life with RA,' I say, feeling the anger move inside me, like a wild horse trying to break out of its box.

'What do you mean?' she asks directly.

Do I tell her how desperate I am? I hesitate, and eventually say, 'I don't want to live. Life seems meaningless. Today is a beautiful day and I want to be outside, rushing around, playing tennis . . . I want to be at Bristol enjoying student life. I can't do what I want to do. I look at my pills and I see a simple way out.' It feels strange to tell a complete stranger this, but natural at the same time.

'How long have you felt this way?'

'I don't know exactly. I think it's been building up for ages.'

'Have you tried to take your life?'

No answer. Another painful silence. But I know she understands the meaning of that silence and I start to cry.

'How do you feel now?' she asks softly, handing me a tissue.

The warm sun shines down on my pale, lifeless face. 'I feel as if it rains all the time, and there's nothing to keep me dry. There's no escape. It just rains and rains and rains . . .'

Session two. I am lying on the sofa bed. 'A friend of mine said the other day, "Oh, you're so lucky to be able to rest all the time and not go to work,"' I tell Jenny. '"People will spoil you so much after the operation too. It's my idea of heaven." I wanted to kill her. Sometimes I feel people don't GET it, how can they be so tactless, so stupid? It was like at Bristol, a girl asked me if I wanted to go skiing with her, nobody really understands. I know I am lucky, I live in a beautiful home, I have a lovely family and friends and there are people far worse off than me. But . . .'

Jenny does not have to say anything. It is just such a release to offload.

Over the next eight sessions we talk about:

1 Illness shame – Bristol and the problems I went
  through in my first term.

2 Tennis, losing my best friend.
3 Vanity – the effects of steroids, the moon face.
4 Insensitive Dr Fischer.
5 The pain coupled with medication which does nothing.
6 The forthcoming hip operation.
7 The stigma attached to arthritis. The misconception that it is only an 'old people's' disease.
8 Friends – Sophie and her support. Finding a way to confide in friends, to open up more.
9 Relationships, boys.
10 Moving on, finding a way forward.

I am crawling out of the mud, I feel stronger mentally. I don't think any of this would have been possible without Jenny's help. I know she can't wave a magic wand and tell me everything will be all right. She does not give me false hope by saying, 'Don't give up, you might be able to play tennis again.' Nor does she say anything intensely irritating like, 'Chin up, be positive.' She understands. She listens patiently, she allows me to hear myself talk. She has made me realize how much pain, anger, frustration and fear is buttoned up inside me, all of it waiting to be released.

She does not offer pat solutions but helps me rationalize things. People won't reject me like a chewed-up tape because I have RA. I still have a purpose – I have a lot to give and also a lot to take out of life. I now believe I can go back to Bristol and not be afraid of telling people, not be afraid to ask for help from friends and tutors. I'm very slowly beginning to shape a new life for myself and I want my new life to be just as good and fulfilling as the old, even if it does contain chronic pain. That will be the difficult part to overcome. The pain. There are no answers, I have to take one day at a time and hope for a miracle drug, a cure. I must never lose sight of hope. Hope will keep me going.

I feel comfortable with Jenny. It did help to talk about wanting to take my life, Mum was right. Why are parents right? It is so irritating.

I'm still scared of the black periods, there will probably be more to come, but at least I know I have someone to talk to. At least I know I can swim to the shallow end again.

It is the end of May and my operation date is drawing near. It has got to the point where the noise in my hip is so unbearable the operation can't happen soon enough.

'I move around like a ninety-year-old, Jenny. Granny can move faster on her stick and she's ninety-three!' I joke. 'When she comes to stay she asks me whether I need a hand and she tells me to sit in the comfy chair while she moves nimbly on to the harder one.' Jenny's face lightens and her mouth breaks into a smile.

'Mum and Helen had to carry me upstairs in a chair the other night and I told Helen she ought to be feeding me grapes at the same time. Mum nearly broke her back and said it was madness, we needed a stair-lift. All I can think about are those dreadful adverts with old people gliding up the stairs at 0.1 miles per hour. You could read a whole book before reaching the top. That will be me! I don't know why I'm still laughing. It's not really funny, is it?'

As I smile, I feel my old self returning. I'm enjoying being out in the sunshine and although being positive will not get rid of my pain, it helps me live with it.

I see Jenny the week before my operation.

'Are you nervous?' she asks.

'No, I was, but I'm beginning to want this operation more than ever. I want to be on my feet again and I want to go back to Bristol next term. My tutor is sending me the reading lists for my History of Art course. He says if I can pass my first year exams I can transfer into the second year. I want to keep up with Sophie, enjoy myself and be with friends again.'

'That's a lot of good wants,' Jenny says, smiling and feeling she has broken through at last.

'I don't think I'll ever "come to terms" with what has happened. I think that's a terrible expression. Why should I *accept* having a crippling disease at my age? Life has dealt me a shit hand but I'm not giving up and I'm going to try to make the most of what lies ahead. I do not want to be a victim, to lie back and let this RA rule my life. I want to fight.'

'The exams and Bristol are something to work towards. When you go back there will still be bad days but . . .'

I cut her off. 'I don't care, I'm going to fight it as hard as I can. It won't beat me.'

33

Bedpans, Thermometers, Needles, Pill Trolleys, Nurse's Charts, Blue Kidney-shape Bowls, Plastic Sheets and Mattresses, Zimmer Frames, Grapes, Plastic Jugs, Ribena, Brown Paper Bag Bins . . .

'Everything off and slip into this,' the nurse says, handing me a white gown.

'Everything?' I ask, mouth wide open. 'Do I have to take my knickers off? Can't they just push them down?'

'Ali, they are doing a hip operation. They are not going to be interested in anything else gubbins, like analysing how beautiful your bottom is,' Helen says.

'I know,' I cough, feeling myself go bright red. 'I just don't like it.' Helen and Mum are laughing at me.

'What about my bra? Why did I have to take that off?' I say to Helen as I am being wheeled away.

'Shut up!'

In the lift on the way down to theatre, my heart beats faster and faster. I am looking forward to the operation. I want to get it over and done with. Any minute now I will be unconscious. Finally I reach the operating theatre and see the surgeon in his blue gown.

'Hi, how are you?' the anaesthetist asks.

'Fine.'

'Good.' A strap is attached to my arm and pads are stuck on to my chest. A needle is injected into my hand for the anaesthetic. I shut my eyes.

'Alice, the anaesthetic is about to go in. Now, I want you to relax, think of somewhere nice.' I am always having to remove myself from my own situation and 'think of somewhere nice'. I am running out of places.

'You'll be asleep before you can even count to five,' he says. This is the bit I've been looking forward to. Surely I can stay awake if I try, I could hold my eyes open. The anaesthetic feels cold.

'One, two . . . three . . . four . . .' I am determined to get to five. Black out.

'Water, I want some water.' I try to sit up. All I can see are distorted figures in blue gowns, all I can hear are footsteps and muffled sounds. Nothing makes sense, my head does not feel attached to my body. I feel disorientated. I feel drunk. This situation feels surreal, abstract, like I'm on a weird planet with aliens walking around me.

'I want to watch TV,' I groan.

'Try to relax, lie back, lie back,' the nurse says, half smiling.

'Where am I? I want my mum. Give me some water.' I feel dizzy and sick and my crusty throat needs watering. 'Why can't I have some water?' I demand, sitting up again.

'You can't have any just yet. Hold on for a bit longer.'

I flop back on to the bed like a rag-doll. 'I need the loo,' I demand crossly.

The nurse slides a bedpan underneath me. It feels as if I am lying on an egg-box.

'She keeps falling asleep on the bedpan,' one of the nurses says fifteen minutes later. 'That can't be comfortable, I wish she'd just go. Alice,' she whispers softly, 'you've fallen asleep again, you obviously don't need to go.'

'Just a little longer,' I say.

'OK,' she smiles.

I pass out again.

I have been given my own room in the ward. Mum looks surprised to see me awake, she had expected me to be totally groggy but instead I am suddenly fully conscious. I keep trying to sit up and the nurse keeps telling me to calm down again. 'Ssh, ssh,' Helen says, looking anxiously at Mum.

A bottle is attached to the wound on my thigh. 'Did it go well?' I ask them.

'Fine,' Mum says. 'You've done so well.'

'I need some water. Water.'

Mum feeds me water like a baby.

'We went shopping and bought you this.' Helen holds up a blue denim shirt. 'It was in the sale, bargain price. We found an old cheap fan to keep you cool in this boiling weather, we also bought you a Walkman because you said you wanted one. Haven't we been spending? I bought myself this too,' she continues nervously, as she holds an Esprit striped top to her chest.

'The pain is getting worse again. It's worse than before,' I cry out.

Helen's face wrinkles, she drops the top and calls a nurse. The nurse looks at my chart. 'She's due to have another shot of morphine, I'll be back in a minute.'

I feel cut up and bruised after being pushed around on the operating table. I feel as if the wound is still exposed.

The top half of the leg they operated on looks as though it has been pumped up to twice the size of my right leg. I suddenly wish I had never EVER said I'd go ahead with the operation. I feel tearful. A part of me has been taken away and it takes the operation to realize how final it is.

'It's sore, it's sore,' I moan.

The nurse injects me with morphine and relief soon floods my body, I shut my eyes and drift in and out of consciousness.

Helen and Mum leave me at about eleven o'clock that evening. Neither really wants to go and Mum knows I'm going to have a restless night.

'Did you get any sleep?' Helen asks the following morning.

'A little. Mum, ring my buzzer. It must be morphine time.'

'I'll go and ask at the desk,' Mum says.

'It hurts,' I sniffle.

'Hang on,' Helen says, stroking my hair gently with her long fingers, the nails painted with purple nail varnish. Her face looks fresh. Her large dark blue eyes and the warmth which radiates from her smile immediately make me feel better. I don't want her to go back to London, back to her graphic design company. She has this incredibly calming presence which envelops you the minute she enters a room.

'There's no morphine on the ward at the moment,' the sister says. 'A nurse is picking some up from another ward. It won't be long, any minute now.'

Half an hour later. 'It still hasn't arrived,' Mum says, frowning at the sister.

An hour later. 'Mum, ask again,' I say frantically. I can't think of anything else. I can't talk to Helen. I need some pain relief and I need it now. I hate being wide awake, in morphine-land my body feels lighter and the pain is numbed, I feel calm, conversations go over my head. I just smile and drift away into oblivion until the numbness begins to disappear, the sharp pain begins to creep in again and consciousness is reawakened . . .

Mum rushes back to the desk while Helen sits close to me. Her aura of calm has become one of frightened panic. 'It's coming,' she reassures me, turning her head to see if Mum is having any luck.

'A nurse will be getting it shortly. She's just gone down now,' the sister repeats.

An hour and a half later. I am angry and desperate. Why are they making my life hell?

The sister sounds like a broken record.

'What's wrong with this ward?' Mum asks, gripping her hair in frustration. 'How can you run out of morphine? I'm sick of being polite!' she shouts, slamming her fist on the table. 'Get the bloody morphine!'

I am counting the days until I can move off my back. Three more days now. The surgeon specified that I must lie on my back for five days and not move at all. I play mindless games like counting the seconds or counting the thousands of tiny pinholes in the ceiling. Life soon becomes a countdown to my morphine jabs; the ward will never run out of it again after the last episode. Receiving mail is another highlight of the day: Dad, who is at home with flu, sends cards almost every day and I know he is with me spiritually. Matthew from Bristol seems to love writing letters on his laptop as he commutes to and from work, he has a summer job to pay off his overdraft.

I try to remember what the next culinary delight will be. Last night I ate chicken fricassee. Then sometimes I wonder what my old, battered hip looked like – what did they do with it? I should have asked if I could see it in a jar. What did the surgeon and his team talk about during the operation? Their shameful bogey or brilliant birdie on the fifth hole? The fire bell rings. If there was a blazing fire enveloping the hospital, how would they get all of us invalids out? The idea of being heaved around makes my heart sink, the simple process of shifting my bottom up and sliding the X-ray film under my hip is an agonizing experience. I suppose we'd be pushed out in our wheely beds, but the old lady opposite is attached to all sorts of contraptions which would surely have to go with her. We are so vulnerable and helpless, our lives are totally in their hands. I hate that feeling. The fire bell is still ringing and I begin to panic, believing my worst nightmare is about to become true, I am going to burn to death.

'No need to panic, false alarm,' I hear one of the nurses saying. 'Don't move, anyone.' What's she talking about? None of us can move anyway.

I model knee-length white granny stockings to stop my blood clotting and Helen paints my toenails bright red to give me something cheerful to look at. She draws patterns on the stockings and sticks a piece of her old chewing-gum on to my little toe.

'Take it off,' I shriek, 'the doctor will be here any minute. Take it off!' I am like a toy Helen can play with.

On day four, my physio, Kate, comes round to see how I am. 'We are going to sit you up early, see if you can walk a little today.'

I want to give it a go but you have to move carefully to prevent the hip dislocating. I can see my scar, which looks neat and healthy, not nearly as vivid, red and angry as I'd imagined. But my leg is still swollen, it does not feel as if it is attached to my body. I try to move. A voice inside my head is saying, 'Don't you dare try to move, I hurt too much.' 'I can't do it, I can't move it any further,' I say, disappointed.

'Right, we'll try tomorrow, give it the full five days,' Kate says, helping me lie back down.

I don't think I'll ever be able to move. I'm scared that something's wrong.

Sophie comes to see me, dressed in pale jeans and a white shirt with a pink cardigan wrapped around her slim waist. Her dark tortoiseshell sunglasses sit on the top of her head, keeping her long hair out of her eyes. She laughs at the antiquated fan Mum and Helen gave me, saying it might fuse the hospital.

She looks tanned and pretty. 'Ali, I know I don't suffer the same pain as you, I can't imagine what it's like.' She starts to bite her lower lip, which is chapped from the sun. 'But I feel as if I've had the operation too. I couldn't concentrate on Thursday because I was thinking of you all day.' I notice tears in her eyes. I have never seen Sophie cry, she is always a shoulder for me to cry on. She bends down to her bag. 'I brought you some jelly babies. And this.' She hands me a tape she has made.

'Best dance hits, great. I suppose I can dance on my crutches.'

'Dance around your zimmer, but it's for when you're grooving on your feet again.'

When Sophie leaves, I wish I could go with her. It is a lovely summer evening and I long to be sitting outside with a beer, laughing and joking with her and my other friends. I think about everything she has said. She shares the sentiments of my parents. They say it is painful watching me suffer, and Mum and Helen might as well have been lying next to me on the operating table while I had the hip operation. It is the same with Sophie, we tackle my illness together: she leads me over the stiles and through the prickly bramble bushes, we get scratched together, and sometimes we get lost, but we always have each other.

The following day Seb visits with a few of his mates. He brings a sponge strawberry cake with whipped cream on the top. Seb and I are good friends again, we have got over the ex-boyfriend awkwardness, but I nevertheless feel embarrassed talking to his friends in my frilly white embroidered nightie and white stockings. I wish I'd had a chance to look in the mirror, to brush my tangled hair and put on a bit of make-up. They have been clubbing all night at the Ministry of Sound and they look spaced out. One of them tells me he took an E tablet for the first time, another tells me he pulled a gorgeous bird. I try desperately to think of something interesting to say, I must keep up, stay cool. I tell them about the morphine.

'You can't get us any, can you?' one of them asks, smiling.

That night I cannot sleep again and decide to watch television. A horror movie is on and one of the male doctors comes into my room and watches it with me. I quite fancy him, but this is no time for romance I think, visualizing bedpans and zimmer frames.

On day five, the thrilling moment arrives – moving from the bed to a chair. I would never have thought that such a move could be so exciting. The pain has eased, although my leg still feels peculiar, as if it does not belong to me. It is wonderful sitting up, and leaving behind those sticky, horrible bed sheets.

I am learning to walk again, it is so strange.

'Right foot forward, now the left,' Kate instructs.

'I can't, it hurts.'

'Come on, you can.'

I feel even more like a granny with my grey zimmer frame. All I need now is a blue rinse. I decide to design young-looking sticks and frames which will feature bright colours and fun patterns, they could even become fashionable accessories too.

Tentatively, I put my left foot down, then my right. I have taken a step. 'At least it doesn't crunch any more,' I say to Kate. This is unbelievable. Not a squeak. I can glide like an ice-skater without a sound.

I am now in a mixed ward, sitting opposite an old lady with a bruised face and grey hair. She loses her temper and lashes out at the nurses all the time. I smile at her but she looks sad; her face is full of expression and yet she never smiles back at me. The boy in the bed next to mine is young. He was bitten by a dog and has a nasty wound.

There is a man on my other side, dressed in a pink T-shirt and silk boxer shorts, who is constantly on the phone. 'Sweet pea, the doctor says I must not, I repeat, must not go back to work for at least another six weeks. Do you think you can manage, petal?' he simpers adoringly. Then he holds one hand over the receiver and with the other angrily slams his cereal bowl back on to the breakfast trolley. 'I asked for wheatflakes, not Weetabix,' he scowls at the long-suffering nurse. 'I must listen to him, petal,' he continues sweetly. After his phone call he stares at me. 'You're a bit young to have had a hip operation, aren't you?' he asks bluntly. 'I know, you're just skiving, you want a holiday,' he laughs. He is not funny and I tell Mum to go and kick him hard in the balls. The man in the bed at the end of the ward broke his leg after falling from his hotel balcony while on honeymoon. He claims he lost his balance and toppled over, but I think he was either drunk, or fighting with his well-endowed bride who pushed him over the rails in a fit of pique . . . the honeymoon already over. 'What do you think?' I whisper to Mum as I reshake the Boggle dice, ready for another game.

'Maybe he was on drugs and thought he could fly,' she says. 'OK, start the time now.' I turn the timer over. 'Stop writing, Alice, I can't see any words yet. Oh lord, do two-letter words count?'

Each day is more positive for me than the last and on day eight I am finally ready for crutches. My leg, very slowly, is beginning to feel part of my body again. I am eager to get going. The sooner I prove I can walk, the quicker I will be able to leave the hospital. That alone is incentive enough.

'Look, Kate, I am almost skipping on my crutches.' Mum claps enthusiastically and dances alongside me as I make my way back to the bed on day nine. I collapse into the chair, laughing until it hurts. The bruised lady is still staring at me, but now I think I can detect a slight interest in her face.

'We will try you on the stairs tomorrow and if you can manage that, then you can be discharged,' Kate says.

On day ten, I receive a bouquet of sunflowers from Sophie, Matthew, Marcus, Rebecca and a few other Bristol friends. Flowers always cheer you up, but I am excited anyway. Today might be the day I leave. I am dying for a fag too. Must leave today.

Discharged! As Mum and I are packing up my things, I look over at the bruised lady again. She is smiling at me. A porter comes to take my luggage and, as I am leaving, I turn around and smile back at her.

Fresh air! Cars! People! Life again. I am so happy to be going home.

It's over.

Medical Update:
I no longer see Dr Fischer. Our last meeting was the best, most productive meeting. I now see one of the leading doctors in research at the Bristol Royal Infirmary. He has put me on to drug Number 8, gold injections. I pray it will prevent further joint damage and disability. I have steroid injections once a month which keep me going, although I know I cannot stay on them permanently. But the most powerful medicine of all is telling people about my condition – tutors, friends. Their support and understanding, more than any pill, makes student life possible.

34

Student Life

October 1995. I'm back at Bristol with my brand new hip. The hip operation was one of the best decisions I have ever made, I can walk without the crunching and I am free from the grating pain. I feel more confident and ready at last to be with other young people.

I'm living in a flat in Clifton with Sophie. There are six of us in all – three boys, three girls. My History of Art tutor, Mr Plant, a kind man with a mole on his round face and a Marlborough Red perpetually hanging out of his mouth, bent over backwards to help me transfer into the second year. He helped me keep up with the course from home by sending lecture notes and reading lists, along with letters asking how I was, which by the end of the summer had lost any trace of formality – we were friendly pen-pals. I was touched by the lengths he went to in helping me prepare for my first-year exams, which I sat in the summer. He has allowed me to keep up with my friends and I'm never going to be left behind again.

I love student life. Our bathroom is damp and smells and my bed comprises two mattresses which sink in the middle, but I don't care. My cooking is uninspiring but I enjoy shopping with Sophie, who helps me reach the boxes of All-Bran or Cup-a-Soup stacked on the highest shelves. I share a cupboard in the kitchen with Marcus and Steven; Marcus's tins are lined up in military fashion compared with my tumbled array of packets of Pasta 'n' Sauce and tins of tuna and Mum's home-made scones, which are often left to mould, much to his disgust. I look forward to the end of lectures, coming home, lighting a fag and opening a bottle of wine. Being in a flat of six, there's always someone around to talk to. The empty wine bottle joins its other friends, lined up on the long table in the hall. The buzzer rings, the telephone rings, music's turned on, we go to the local pubs, we organize house parties. We have fun and at last I feel like an ordinary student, studying for my degree. Each day is an achievement of my independence.

My flatmates are wonderful, they are on hand when I need help. They fetch me hot-water bottles, undo tight lids, buy bags of frozen peas to put on my knees – Sophie and I even eat them frozen too! They give me an arm for support, they talk to me at my bedside if I'm having a bad day, carry heavy books for me. The last two and a half years have brought Sophie and me closer than we've ever been. We work our way around problems together and perhaps that's one good thing which can be said for having any kind of illness – it can show you who your friends are and strengthen those friendships to a level you never knew existed.

I'm also loving my work. I have two new tutors – the head of the History of Art Department, Mr Burness, and Mrs Wickham, who teaches me Design and Applied Arts. Both are fully aware of my situation but they don't single me out or make me feel different from the rest of the class, and if I need to catch up on missed tutorials or lectures they offer help in private. One of my flatmates and I are planning a trip to Venice to see the Titians and Bellinis. Up until my course began I had hardly set foot in a gallery or museum – and although a complete contrast to playing tennis in America, I am enjoying my course far more than I imagined and it's wonderful to have a different challenge.

'Ali, I've had a shit morning, my politics assignment is driving me mad,' Sophie says, plonking her file on the kitchen table.

'Bath? Lunch?' I suggest, grinning. If either of us is stressed we take my car out and often end up in Bath, our favourite shopping haven. I know the shops back to front and inside out. 'Let's go to that Spanish bar where they give you loads of olives and bread.'

She gives me a disapproving look. 'I ought to stay and work, finish the essay.' Sophie is conscientious and highly motivated.

Sophie and I are picking at the olives and bread. 'How's Tom?' she asks fondly.

'He's still with the community in Wales. He's quite happy but he's picked up really odd phrases, probably from the other inmates.'

'Like what?' she smiles, stirring her Diet Coke with a straw.

'His latest is, "A man's wallet is his own kingdom."'

'What's happened to "How much for the gun?" Or "ride 'em high, Billy Ray?"' she asks, wrinkling her nose in amusement.

'He hasn't said that for a while. He mutters "keep calm" a lot too.'

'I'd love to understand how his mind works. I sometimes wish I was still reading psychology,' Sophie says.

'Mum told me she was at Sainsbury's the other day and

Tom said to the man behind the fish counter, "Don't serve my mum, she's from the Mafia!" And then every time she asked for some prawns or cod or whatever, Tom was saying, "Greedy guzzgog, greedy guzzgog." How would you analyse that?!'

We both laugh. 'Hey, change the subject, it's your twenty-first soon, you must have a party,' Sophie says excitedly. 'Let's make a list.' We scribble names down on our paper napkins, laughing as we pair up the most unlikely couples.

Later that evening, with well-cleansed faces and wearing stripy pyjamas, we sit on Sophie's bed talking until the early hours of the morning.

'Bed,' I say eventually, getting up to leave. 'Night.' As I am closing her door I hear a muffled voice from under the duvet, 'Al, you know you are one of the most important people in my life.'

'You are too,' I say, quietly shutting her door.

It's 25 January, my twenty-first birthday. Mum and Dad take me and my flatmates out for lunch as a thank-you for all they do for me as well as a birthday celebration. Later, Mum kisses me goodbye and says, 'You look more like the old Alice than you have done in nearly three years.' Her voice wavers with emotion. I watch from the window of our flat as my parents drive away. Dad is beeping the horn furiously. Mum turns to wave, tears flowing down her cheeks.

In the evening I have a fondue party and Helen comes down. She tells me all about her new boyfriend, James, and I can tell by the way she is talking that she is already in love.

I seat Rebecca next to me as I haven't seen her for ages. We drink sea-breezes and round off the night with tequilas. I throw up on Matt's shoe.

Helen and I sleep head to toe. 'Helen?' I sit up.

'Um,' she mutters, half asleep.

'When I leave Bristol I want to go to London like you, like everyone else, and get a job. I can do it, can't I?'

'Of course you can, my darling, of course you can.'

'And I'd love to meet someone,' I say. 'I will meet someone, won't I?'

'I know you will.'

'I should be sharing my bed with a handsome young man, not you.'

'Go to sleep, you cheeky monkey!' She turns over.

I lay my head on the pillow, knowing I'll have a terrible hangover but feeling happy and looking forward to the next day.

35

Blind Date

'Alice, phone, it's Matthew,' Sophie calls from the bottom of the stairs. Everyone chipped in for a portable BT phone, mainly for me to keep upstairs so that I don't have to go up and down like a yo-yo.

'Thanks for the fondue party the other night,' Matt says.

'Your shoes,' I squeak, having an embarrassing flashback. 'I got far too drunk, I'm so sorry.'

'I don't care about my shoes,' he laughs. 'They didn't cost me two hundred pounds like yours! Anyway, how about dinner soon at my place, I make a wicked lasagne.'

'OK, cool.'

'Great, come round tonight, seven-thirty.'

'Do you want me to bring anything?'

'Just yourself, darling,' he says. 'That's enough for me.'

'Ugh, you smooth talker.'

'When I'm going out with someone I always think the grass is greener on the other side of the fence. But,' Matthew says, pouring me another glass of wine, 'when I get to the other side there's always a drought, and I find myself standing in a field of dried weeds with a few measly dead-looking flowers.' He takes a drag on his joint and passes it to me. 'Does grass help the pain?'

'Yes, makes me feel relaxed.' I inhale deeply. 'Carry on, back to your story.'

'Yes, to go back to the other grass . . .'

'The weeds,' I tease.

'Why is it so hard to find someone you click with?'

'Matthew, you are always going out with someone. What are you looking for?'

'Someone I feel comfortable with, whom I can say anything to . . .'

'I've been asked out by someone,' I say. 'We're going out tomorrow.'

'Oh?' Matthew looks at me. 'Who is he? Why haven't you told me about him before?'

'Don't sound so surprised and don't use the Marcus "He must be deaf and blind" joke.'

'Who is he?' Matthew repeats.

'He's called Josh. I hardly know him so there's nothing to tell.'

'Yet,' he smiles, pulling the cork out of another bottle of wine.

I met Josh at a party, we talked, and the next day we bumped into each other at Boots, along the shampoo aisle. He asked whether I would meet him for a drink later in the week. I am flattered, but I am also very nervous. It's like a blind date, we may have nothing in common and he doesn't know I have rheumatoid arthritis – I'm going to have to tell him. I am not going to lie. If he likes me, he likes me, and if he doesn't like me because of my RA then it's too bad. He's good-looking – short, dark hair brushed to the front and sleepy brown eyes.

*

'You are lovely,' Josh says, looking into my sparkling eyes. He pulls the band from my hair – long, golden brown locks fall around my shoulders.

'You should wear it down more often,' he says, twisting my hair, playing with it in his hands. He lights some tall scented candles. His lovely face glows in the subdued light. He reaches over for the champagne glasses and we both take a sip. He slowly, teasingly, plays with the buttons of my cardigan. With each one that he undoes, he kisses me on my bare stomach, sending shivers of excitement down my spine. He is a smooth operator. I can't take my eyes off him! He gently eases my top off. 'You've got beautiful soft skin,' he murmurs, kissing my shoulders. His warm hands are around my waist and then his hands move back to my face, he strokes my cheeks and we kiss again. One hand begins to play with the tie of my trousers and I slip out of them quickly. I'm wearing my silk Calvin Klein knickers with matching bra; I have thought this out immaculately, to the last detail, I think proudly. I am oozing sex and I know he wants me. I pull Josh towards me and we kiss passionately. His lips are covered in my red lip gloss.

'You taste like strawberries,' he says, and, like a wild beast pouncing on its prey, he scoops me up into his hairy, masculine arms and leads me to his bed. The water gurgles beneath me. Thrilling! I've always wanted to do it in a waterbed, ever since watching the film, *Women in Red* with Kelly Le Brock.

He feeds me more champagne, licking the bubbles all over my naked body. He takes his clothes off and I throw my knickers and bra on to the floor, cooing like an excited monkey. We both giggle in nervous anticipation . . .

*

'Alice, phone,' Sophie says, 'It's Josh.'

I am lying at the end of my bed, one leg hanging over the side, the sheets halfway down my body. One of the buttons has fallen off my nightshirt. Why did Sophie have to spoil it just when I was coming to the juicy part? 'Hi,' I say, pulling myself together.

'Hi, just checking we're still on for the pub tonight?'

'Yes, I'll pick you up,' I say, a flutter of nerves. I can see myself going red. Does he know I've been dreaming, fantasizing about him? I feel almost guilty.

I have been grappling with the handbrake for the last ten minutes. I am cursing Sophie who drove the car last and forgot to leave it on low. I am groaning with frustration. 'Will you please go down, you stupid handbrake, please. I'm going to be late,' I shout at it. A stranger walks past and I open the window. 'Oh excuse me, excuse me,' I plead desperately at his retreating back. He turns around. 'I'm having a bit of a problem,' I say. 'I can't release the handbrake down.'

'I'm sorry?' he asks incredulously.

'I have arthritis, my hands, I can't do it,' I stutter, verging on tears.

He gets into the passenger seat and releases it in one simple manoeuvre. 'There you are,' he says softly. I thank him profusely and begin my journey to Josh's flat.

There are no parking spaces near his flat so I beep the horn loudly outside his door, praying he'll know it's me. I am blocking the road and I'll be facing road-rage soon. Hurry up. Josh skips down the steps; he's wearing Levis, a rugby shirt and cap. He looks gorgeous as he throws open the door. 'Hi,' he smiles, kicking the Diet Coke cans and tape boxes to one side. I had planned to give my car a clean before the turmoil of the handbrake incident made me forget. He picks up my orange disabled discs.

I snatch them from him before he has a chance to see my name. 'Oh, fancy that, hey? Must be . . . Mum's, she's always leaving them in my car by mistake!' Mum's? I could have done better than that. What's happened to my 'Let's tell the truth, no more lies' motto?

'What's wrong with your mum?' he asks.

'She has tennis elbow,' I bluff.

'My grandfather has those discs,' Josh says. 'Poor old man, he recently had a hip operation. It takes him nearly an hour to get in and out of his car, let alone drive it. He still manages though. Amazing old man.'

'Yeah, really brave,' I say.

'When I see him I feel so lucky to be young, it really sinks in you know, being slow and cranky would drive me insane.'

'Um,' I mutter under my breath, wanting the date to end here and now.

'Aren't you glad to be young and fit, to be at university?'

'It's great,' I say, smiling radiantly. Lying is so much easier than the truth. Well, I am young and I am at university . . .

I manage to park right outside the pub. Josh gets the drinks while I go to the loo and lean against the wall. I must tell him. Tell him, you idiot.

'One vodka and tonic for you, madame,' he says as I sit back down at the table.

'So, tell me all about you,' I say. That's it, just focus

the conversation on him. Boys love talking about them-selves, don't they? And he is lovely, I'm sure he's interesting.

'And you?' Josh says eventually, after spending the entire evening talking about his music career. He plays the guitar.

'Last orders,' the barman calls.

'I think it's time to leave,' I smile, relief flooding my body. 'I'm quite tired.'

We arrive at his flat. 'Come in, for a coffee at least,' he says.

I haven't got my pills, I will be in agony if I stay the night without my steroids to keep me going and I won't be able to move at all the following morning. My knee is swollen at the moment too. God, it makes me so angry that I have to consider these things. I would love to spend the night with him. I want to be carefree like I used to be. Hang on, it's just a coffee. 'Yes, that's fine,' I hear myself saying.

Josh plays some of his music while I sit on his sofa drinking Bailey's. A coffee never means a coffee, does it? But I'm happy listening to him play, he's really good, sounds like Tom Petty. 'Can you play, "Free fallin'"', by Tom Petty?'

He puts the guitar down. 'I know who it's by,' he smiles, walking over. We start to kiss, his lips feel lovely. I want to be touched. My fears are disappearing. Suddenly I pull away, smiling.

'What's so funny?' he asks.

'Nothing,' I reassure him, 'it's just this dream I had the other night.'

'So nothing to do with me then, I haven't got some-thing stuck in my teeth or . . .'

'No. It's not you, promise.'

'Good.' He plays with my shirt and pulls my shoulders up, it hurts, one crunches. 'What was that noise?' he asks.

'Nothing,' I say quickly. 'I need the loo.' I get up, knocking the bottle of Bailey's on to the floor. 'Oh God, sorry,' I say, picking it up. Luckily it's empty. I lock the door and take the shirt off myself. Underneath I'm wearing a simple vest top, easier to slip off, and thank goodness for drawstring trousers. Stop! Alice, you're being a fool, you must tell him. Why are you so scared to tell him – fear of rejection? Remember what Mum says: 'I must not hide behind my illness, must not be ashamed.' I know she's right. Matthew, Marcus, Helen, Rebecca and Sophie say the same. But this is only our first date and I can't get all heavy, I need to get to know him before I can tell him. Alice! He'll find out anyway, there's only so much covering up you can do, so tell him! No, I must leave, I can see him another time. 'How am I going to get out of this?' I think, panicking. No, I'll stay. I need to know that I can still be attractive, wanted. But it's not really me if I'm hiding one major part of my life, is it? I keep changing my mind. Eventually I go back, trying to look refreshed and at ease. I sit next to him. We kiss again. We walk to his bedroom.

My heart sinks when I see that it's a futon bed on the floor. His CDs, records and lecture notes are scattered across the sheets, a dirty coffee mug is next to the bed, along with a half-eaten piece of toast and Marmite. My eyes scan the bed with fear. How will I get on to it? Suddenly I wish I was with someone like Matthew. I feel comfortable with him, he would help me down, and we could have a joke about it too. God, I wish I fancied him, but I don't. It's always the way.

'Sit down,' Josh says, tidying his bed.

I manoeuvre myself in a totally unorthodox way, crashing down on to my knees like a fat elephant and swivelling around on my bottom. I can feel bruises creating patterns on my knees.

'Are you all right there?' he asks, hearing the thud of me landing on the mattress.

'Fine,' I shriek unnaturally, while all I can think about is how I am going to get up again. Desperately, I look around for anything I might be able to use to pull myself up. 'Let's put some music on,' I say brightly.

He leaps up and puts on a track. Why can't I have normal knees and normal arms to pull myself up with?

'Come a bit closer,' he says, pulling my shoulders again. 'What is that noise?'

'What noise?' I ask, my voice rising.

He pulls me on top of him and the weight on my elbows is straining my arms and shoulders. I can feel the discomfort in every joint. I am so nervous, my body has seized into spasm and I can't move. I feel like a block of lard lying on top of him. Suddenly I have sobered up very quickly. My shoulders are trembling.

'You're shaking,' he says. 'What's wrong?'

I move away from him. There is a terrible, awkward silence. 'I need a hand up,' I say eventually. I can't go through with this, I can't.

'What?'

'Help me up, please,' I say, holding my top protectively around my body. 'I've got to go.'

'What's wrong?' he asks again. 'Don't go, I really want you to stay.'

'Please,' I repeat, close to tears.

'I'm sorry.'

'No, I'm sorry, it's not your fault. I've got rheumatoid arthritis. I should have told you, I . . . look, it hurts, my shoulder hurts, my knees . . . I can't explain. If you're still interested give me a call and I can tell you more. Just not now. I have to go.'

Josh does not call. I have learnt Mum's lesson the hard way.

36

Conflicts

I am sitting in the clinic at Bristol Royal Infirmary. It took me nearly an hour to park and I have been here for over an hour waiting to have my gold injection. The beginning of my third year has been terrible. I am no longer being given steroid drips because the doctor worries about the damage to my bones. The RA has reared its ugly head again, it's been let free to invade my body with its usual relentless aggression. The gold is useless, but there is little else to try and my doctor and I are pulling at desperate straws. Finally I get back to the flat, slamming the door behind me. A ten-second jab of nothingness has taken up my entire morning again. My anger has reached boiling point, it is like hot milk in a pan waiting to spill over the edge.

Work fills a vital gap when I am unable to lead a full student life. It preserves my sanity. Ideas for my dissertation, presenting talks with slides, thoughts on my Design and Applied Arts or Modern British Art essays – work gets me up in the mornings and it gives me a purpose. Sophie tells me my room looks like a chaotic library when she hands me two more books she collected for me earlier. I am still in bed, buried under the rubble of books, files and paper with ink all over my fingers and my hair like a bird's nest. She laughs, saying I look as though I could do with a break. We have a coffee together.

'Alice, really,' she says more seriously, 'this has gone on for too long. You can't continue like this. You need to go back on the steroids.'

'But I can't, they're more harmful in the long run.'

'But look at you now!' she exclaims.

'Soph, mornings are always worse,' I say, trying to reason with her and myself. 'I'll be fine. Anyway, I'm going home later.' I am forced to divide my time between home and Bristol and my independence is trickling away again, like water through a plughole.

'Oh, hi, Mr Burness, I'm sorry but I can't come in to see you about my essay today,' I say, sprawled on my bed half-dressed. 'I'm feeling awful, I think I'm going to go home.'

'I'm sorry you're not too good,' he says awkwardly. Mr Burness rarely asks me questions about the RA; I'm sure it makes him feel uneasy but I can sense his understanding. 'You did well with your essay, Alice, it was the Whistler one wasn't it?'

'Yes. How exactly did I do?' I ask, perking up immediately.

'How about I come to you?' he suggests.

'This is a nice flat,' Mr Burness remarks, sitting at the kitchen table. I look at him anxiously as he reads over his comments on my essay. He is a wonderful teacher and tutor – he has been teaching for many years and can make any subject interesting. He could talk about the dullest artist and still leave you feeling inspired. 'I really enjoyed this,' he says warmly, handing me back my work. I look relieved. 'You mustn't worry, Alice. Where are we now?' he mutters to himself. 'Something like twelve weeks until finals. It's Easter soon . . .' His eyes light up at the thought of a break. 'You're doing very well and remember that your second-year exams count towards your finals and you got a high 2.1.' He takes off his little round glasses and wipes his eyes. 'And I can lend you this book for your dissertation. It's a rare edition so please look after it,' he stresses, as he lifts an old bound book on Impressionism out of a carrier bag.

'I have been trying to get a copy of this for ages. Oh God, thank you so much.'

He runs a hand through his hair. 'If you can't get access to some of the books you need, ask me. I know what it's like, the library never has enough copies and I don't mind lending them to students, as long as they don't come back with coffee stains on them. Right,' he says, rising. 'I must be off.'

'Thanks for coming over. You are always so kind,' I say, hearing myself gush.

'It was fine. It kept me from the bar for another hour, which is a good thing too,' he smiles. He notices my overnight bag resting against the front door. 'Make the most of your time at home, get plenty of rest and don't come back until you're up to it.' The deep-set lines in his forehead show his concern, but I feel dreadful all the time – whether I rest or not. If I'd taken his advice, I'd never have gone to Bristol.

'You'll do well, Alice, you deserve to leave with a good degree.' I smile back at him, grateful for his reassurance. Getting my degree is not just about me – I want to give Mr Burness something back too.

I've got to get through my last term.

One more week until the Easter break. Sophie is at my bedside, she hands me a hot-water bottle. Steven tries to sit me up in bed and I wince. Every movement is raw, the debilitating pain shoots through my body.

'It'll wear off soon,' I say, trying to reassure Sophie, whose face is lined like a creased linen shirt. 'Have you rung Mum?' I ask her.

She hands me a drink with a straw. 'Yes, she's picking you up later this morning.'

I look at my unopened books. Deadlines for essays and dissertations are creeping up too quickly and I am missing valuable days of work.

Steven and Marcus help Mum carry me downstairs and into the car. I watch the anxious faces of Sophie and my flatmates fade into the distance as Mum and I head home.

My five flatmates, and Sophie in particular, don't know how they are going to cope with both helping me and revising for their finals. We should have talked about this earlier. Finals are in eight weeks time and I am having too many flare-ups, it's not surprising they're worried. I'm worried. My doctor has put me on a higher dose of steroid to help me get through the last term but I hate being on steroids, they are the final resort. I will do anything to hold on to the last shred of independence I have.

I need to be surrounded by people who are also doing finals, feel I am a part of the process. I cannot be at home all the time, cut off completely. Ideally I would like to be in Bristol for two nights a week because I still have tutorials. Rachael, an old family friend whom I adore, lives fifteen minutes away from the flat, and tells me she will be on stand-by if I need her. She has been a great ally in Bristol, often taking me to doctor's appointments, or having me to stay when I need a rest and proper food. She looked after us when we were babies and has remained part of the family ever since.

My parents speak to Sophie's mother at the beginning of our final term; they all agree that me spending two nights a week in the flat is a reasonable plan.

I do not expect my flatmates to be there for me twenty-four hours a day. I tell Sophie to shut her door, get on with her work, and not feel guilty. If I can't manage, I'll ring home.

It's the second week of term, and I'm at home with my nose buried in a file in my bedroom. Steven rings. 'Alice, we need to talk to you. We're worried about you,' he begins apprehensively.

'What do you mean?'

He hesitates. 'Well, what with finals and everything, we are all under an immense amount of pressure and we don't think we'll be able to manage if you have a bad day, we couldn't be there for you.'

'Steven ,we've been through all of this.'

'Yes, but the first week was not as we had planned, you should have sorted out seeing your tutor earlier. You came up on Monday, not Wednesday . . .'

I cut him off. 'I know, I'm sorry.'

'Well, it's not just that . . . We are worried that if you are not well we won't be able to concentrate. Every minute is valuable.'

'Well, why are you are wasting time worrying when we have talked about this already?'

'But,' he stammers, 'we are not happy.'

'What are you trying to say? That I can't come up to the flat at all?'

'It's just, well, what if Thursday is bad? We would feel so bad leaving you in your room knowing you were in pain while we were just getting on with our work.'

'Steven, I wish I could guarantee that everything will be fine but I can't. Work in the library if you are so worried, I don't want you to be there for me. I promise that Rachael will be around if I need her. And my parents. I'll only drive up on Wednesday if I'm feeling all right anyway.'

'But what if you're bad on Thursday? We can't take any risks,' he says firmly.

'I'll ring Rachael immediately,' I say despairingly. 'Finals aren't easy and my illness is unpredictable. You've been so supportive in the past but I do not expect anything from you during the exams. We've got to be strong and get on with it, whether I'm bad or not.'

'Well, what if Rachael is not there?'

'But she lives fifteen minutes away. She knows she may be needed for those two days a week, she's putting them aside.'

'We just do not feel comfortable with this. We feel in a way that we have done so much for you, it's sort of your turn now to help us out a bit,' Steven says uneasily.

'You want me to vanish into thin air until finals are over? I won't be able to see friends, or go to my last tutorials, or the library,' I swallow hard, almost in tears.

'But we can send you any work or books you need.'

'Well, you've made it pretty clear I'm not welcome, so

fine, get on with your work. I won't be coming to the flat at all, not even for two measly days.'

I am furious. They can have their way but I am not going to be gracious about it. I think they are being grossly unfair. They, too, think I am being grossly unfair and they feel hard done by. We are suddenly miles apart, on totally different wavelengths.

I talk to my parents. Dad is angry and upset for me. He can see that by cutting me off they are hurting me enormously; but on a practical level, he is *paying* for me to be in the flat and they are saying I cannot be there. Five minutes later the phone rings again. It is Sophie.

'I think you are being selfish, Sophie.'

She is insulted. 'I can't believe you think we want to hurt you after everything we've been through,' she says defensively, 'but it's finals and ultimately we are here to get a degree.'

'We are all here to get a degree! It's not just you taking finals! I know you don't want to hurt me but you are, whether you want to or not. I can't be at home all the time. I need to have a little normality.'

'But you have to accept it, you're *not* normal like us.' There is silence. How can she say this? She has thrust the knife in and twisted it a thousand times. 'After everything we have done for you, it is our turn to ask for help. Please, Alice, we need this time to work, it's only eight weeks. We'll still be in touch. Ali,' she pleads, 'please don't take it personally, it's only because of finals, once they're over everything will go back to normal.'

'After everything we have done for you' – it's them and me. I feel like a freak, a charity case, an alien, an outsider.

This is what upsets me. I cannot deny that without their support Bristol would have been impossible for me, but it feels as if they have been clocking up these favours. In return I must do them the gigantic favour of not existing during 'their' finals. I should not mind doing this because I should be enormously grateful for 'everything they have done for me'. I thought I had been a friend to them and I would do anything for any of them, in particular Sophie. But what they are asking of me doesn't seem right, it puts a different set of values on our relationship.

Our friendship, the closeness, the trust, the support, the love, the care, and the fun we have all shared together has been destroyed. My friendship with Sophie is shattered to smithereens, like a precious glass bowl broken into hundreds of tiny pieces.

I drive up for my tutorial with Mr Burness and then drive to see Mrs Wickham, my Design and Applied Arts teacher, at her home. Mrs Wickham often organizes group student suppers or lunches at her house, which is like a museum, full of beautiful clocks, antiques and pictures. After burrowing around in her attic room, finding useful revision books, we walk back down the creaky stairs into the kitchen. In the midst of going over exam papers we go off on a slight tangent, sharing nostalgic memories of the past year. She tells me what some of her old pupils are doing now and her face lights up when she talks about them – the devoted attention Mrs Wickham gives to each of her pupils is overwhelming. She supports and encourages us all right to the end and beyond. She asks me what I would like to do. Mid-sentence, I break down; suddenly I can't help telling her what's happened in the flat and I can hear myself talking really quickly and not making any sense.

'Tell me slowly,' she interrupts warmly but firmly. 'Come on, what's happened? Start again.' Mrs Wickham listens without taking sides. I tell her that I probably won't get to her few remaining lessons.

'It doesn't matter, we can go through the last tutorials now. Tell Mr Burness too, he will understand,' she assures me. 'It's not the first time there have been dramas during finals. It's a very stressful period at the best of times, Alice, for everyone concerned. Try not to let this get in the way.'

'I will, I've got no excuse now,' I smile, looking at the pile of books she has found for me.

At four o'clock, all the clocks dotted around the house start chiming and she laughs. 'Keep in touch. I'm here all the time, just call me. OK, a cup of tea and then back to work?'

When I finally leave I feel much better. Talking to her was like talking to a very good friend.

When I'm not driving up and down to Bristol, I work in my bedroom at home, but it is at night that the argument with the flatmates haunts me. I can't believe it's happened. I feel miserable, hurt and let down. I feel sad. I miss them all enormously, but when I remember what Steven and Sophie said, I feel so angry again. I have an uneasy feeling that it won't be resolved, and notions of not wanting to carry on, of giving up and taking my life, start to creep back. Without friends, what's life worth, what's left?

Helen comes down for the weekend and talks it through with me. She is a strong shoulder to cry on.

I'm six weeks through the term and finals are imminent. I'm at home all the time now. It's a Monday afternoon, I am in my bedroom working with Jasmine, my faithful little companion, sitting at my feet. I hear her gnawing away at the chair and tell her to stop. I look down and see a corner of the precious book given to me by Mr Burness chewed up with sharp little teeth marks. 'No,' I cry out in despair. 'Fuck fuck, FUCK!' I scream, dreading having to tell him. Can anything else go wrong, I think, collapsing on to my bed. Jasmine looks up at me with innocent eyes. The phone rings. She growls and yanks the receiver off the hook. 'Bugger off, you stupid animal,' I yell.

'Alice, is that you. Alice?'

I pick up the phone. 'Hello,' I say, out of breath.

'Alice, hi, where have you been? What's going on?' I can hear amusement in her voice. It's Rebecca. 'I called for you at the flat and they told me you were at home. Why are you at home? I wanted to meet for a drink.'

Rebecca is a lovely friend. We can go for weeks without talking to one another, but when we meet it's like we spoke yesterday, our friendship never changes. I tell her straight away. I am not going to pretend that I am at home out of choice.

'I can't believe it. I'm going over there right now to give them a piece of my mind. You can't stay at home the whole time. Let me go and talk to them.'

'If you want to,' I say, deeply touched, although I doubt it will change things.

Rebecca talks to Marcus.

'Well, you have never *lived* with Alice, you don't know how ill she is sometimes,' he tells her.

'But she doesn't expect to be in the flat seven days a week. Surely it's not too much for you all? How would you feel if you weren't allowed to be in your own flat?'

'Well, I have to support Sophie. She's the one Alice leans on the most. With finals she just can't cope.'

I tell Mum about Rebecca's support. Mum, up until now, has been quiet about the situation. 'You do think I'm right, don't you?' I say to her, longing for reassurance.

'There is no right or wrong, but I think we should have organized something much earlier for you. I should have seen this coming,' she confesses.

'But how could . . .' I start to argue.

'Rebecca is a great friend,' she says, stopping me in my tracks, 'but she does not know what goes on behind the scenes, what the dreadful days are really like. I should have been more aware that Sophie and the others were finding it difficult, and with the added pressure of finals . . .'

I look at Mum as if she's the enemy.

'Alice, it is one of the most heart-wrenching things watching someone you love suffer and not being able to help them. Yes, you're the one in terrible pain, but we feel it too. It can't have been easy for Sophie. Remember that.'

I'm working, working, working. I am making up for lost time. But, most importantly, work is a great distraction. It takes my mind off the situation.

I miss Sophie terribly. I lie awake at night, hugging the

brown fluffy dog she gave me, its ear soaked with my tears. Self-doubt creeps in. Of course they're not malicious and I know they don't want to hurt me. Am I being fair to them? Should I have accepted gracefully that they needed this chunk of time on their own? The first week did not work out exactly as we had planned because I was seeing my tutor . . . but I should have been rigid in my plans. Was I naïve to believe that Sophie would not worry? Sophie wasn't clocking up favours, it just became too much, she was emotionally drained and I didn't see it. I have been blinkered and selfish. Should I swallow any pride left and try to make it up with them? No friendship is worth losing, is it? Especially the one Sophie and I have built up together over the years. But maybe it is too late . . .

I hate taking my exams and not seeing her friendly face afterwards. We used to talk about our exams together over a glass of wine and a cigarette. We would laugh about the subjects we had spent hours revising and which had not come up at all in the paper.

I now fear bumping into my flatmates and I'm sure they feel the same as me. It is like walking around on eggshells. After my Design and Applied Arts exam, a crowd of us walk to Browns. I spot Sophie walking down the steps but she does not see me. She looks dreadful, tired and even thinner than usual. I know I have hurt her too.

'The way you talk about your friendship, it would be a great shame to let this come between you,' Jenny says softly. Her counselling has been invaluable since the break-up with the flatmates. 'But you can only work it out when you are both ready. I think your friendship is strong enough to pick up the pieces eventually.' She half smiles. 'This is a dreadful cliché, Alice, but time heals.'

At home, the night before my last exam, Sophie rings. It is a total surprise, as we have not talked for eight weeks now. 'I wanted to wish you good luck,' she says.

'This whole situation, I hate it,' I say, happy to hear her voice.

'Me too. Let's meet after your final exam?'

'I'd love to.'

We walk slowly to a café up the road and order two cappuccinos. I hope we can put everything behind us but when I speak to Sophie again, I realize we have both hurt each other too much. The gap between us has grown wider and deeper. Our feelings are too raw to even begin trying to reconcile them.

Later, I ring Matthew and take a bottle of wine to his place and stay the night. We sit on his terrace, wrapped in sleeping-bags. Matthew makes me laugh and cry at the same time.

I can't sleep. I creep down the stairs and find Matthew still awake.

'It's not worth it,' he says, noticing my tears. He puts an arm around me. 'You should be celebrating after the exams, not feeling miserable.' He's right.

The following morning I go to see Rebecca.

'Alice, hi. God you look awful,' she says, taking my bag. 'Are you OK?'

After telling her what's happened, she says I can stay with her for as long as I want. We have two weeks to wait for our results and we go out to celebrate our finals being over. Rebecca and I become very close, we make tentative plans to live together in London and talk about going on a summer holiday. Rebecca makes me feel less vulnerable and alone.

Her friendship saves me.

37

Results

The day of our results has come. Rebecca and I are eating lunch outside in Clifton. The sun burns against my back. I want to prolong lunch for as long as I can – the prospect of ringing Mr Burness to hear my results is terrifying.

I also feel on edge because I have to go to the flat to collect my things for good. I want to go today, get it over with.

'Are you sure you don't want me to come with you?' Rebecca asks.

'No.'

'Do you think you can patch things up?'

'I don't know.'

I still have my key to the flat. I creep up the stairs and through the front door. Marcus is watching television. He gets up to go to the kitchen and walks past, totally ignoring me, so I go upstairs to my bedroom. The mobile which normally sits recharging is not there. I can hear Sophie talking. When she has finished, I go to her room and knock on the door. I never used to knock politely on her door. I am really nervous, which strikes me suddenly as absurd. There is a moment of awkward silence before I ask her if I can use the phone.

Like a stranger she hands it to me.

Back in my bedroom. My back is hurting, I kick off

my shoes. It takes at least another ten minutes before I pluck up the courage to call the History of Art department.

'Alice, hi, you're the last to call. Mr Burness has been longing to speak to you,' the secretary says.

'Oh?' I ask hopefully.

'I can't say anything. I'll put you through.' I can sense her smiling.

Mr Burness comes on the line. 'Alice, congratulations. You got a First. The Examination Board did not even have to take your case into account.'

'I can't believe it!' I say incredulously.

'It was a remarkable effort. I'm so pleased for you.'

'I wish I was there so I could hug you,' I tell him emotionally.

'Well, come and see me. I'd love that,' he laughs.

Next, I ring home. 'Mum, it's me. I got a First,' I whisper.

Mum has been in the garden pulling out weeds – anything to take her mind off waiting for a call from me. She's crying.

Downstairs the flatmates are watching television. None of them turns their head. I want to share my news, hug Sophie, ask her how she did, ask the others how they did. I want to go out and celebrate with them as if nothing had happened. I wish I could tell Sophie how much I miss her. I want things to be the way they were, but something inside me just cannot say sorry.

All I can think of to say is, 'Oh, I see we've got new sofas in the sitting-room.'

'Yep,' one of them shrugs, and carries on eating.

I go back up to my room. I am not welcome.

The phone rings. It's Mrs Wickham congratulating me.

'Hug yourself with pride,' she says. Her words make me feel so high, similar to when I won an exciting tennis match. I didn't think I'd ever feel like this again.

Who can I call now? I'm longing to talk to someone. I ring Matthew and then ring Helen. She is at a work leaving-do party. It is about half past three and she is plastered. 'Alice, everyone wants to talk to you,' she says, almost in tears. Before I have the chance to say no, I am talking to someone from her office, equally pissed.

'Hi, this is Grant. I hear you got a First. Your sister really loves you, you know. She's been telling me all about you,' he slurs. 'I'm going to pass you on to John now, he wants a word with you.'

'Everyone wants a word with you,' I can hear Helen shrieking in the background. 'Did you know my sister got a First?' she is saying around the table. I can hear cheers. I feel so happy. I wish I could join their party. Finally, I am passed back to Helen after speaking to virtually the entire company. 'You must go out and celebrate tonight. Where are you now?' she asks.

'In the flat.'

'Why? I thought you were staying with Rebecca.'

'I am. Oh, I don't know, I should never have come here.'

'Look, it's the best news I've had in ages. Go and get seriously drunk and forget about it all.'

I begin to collect everything that belonged to me – CDs lying around the flat, cookery books, my mobile phone, posters off the wall.

I slip out of the flat with my things. They are still watching television. Sophie and I catch each other's eye as I quietly shut the door behind me. I will never forget her friendship and I hope that maybe we can be friends again. She gave me so much and I hope I gave her something back in return.

I walk slowly to my car, wishing with all my heart that I could run. If I did not have rheumatoid arthritis I would be skipping across the park, screaming at everyone that I got a First. Well, I cannot run but my heart skips instead.

38

The Trial: Part 2

I am sitting in the front of the conference hall with Dr Campbell.

'You need some new folders for my notes,' I suggest, looking at their torn, tatty front covers. Paper is bulging out of each of the three medical files.

'Yes, I know. I need a trolley to wheel them around too,' he smiles. 'Are you feeling all right? Ready to face them all?'

I nod. I've been dreaming about this moment for a long time and don't wish to be anywhere else.

The trial for this new drug has been all I can think about for weeks. It's an anti-TNF drug. TNF stands for 'tumour necrosis factor', an inflammatory molecule, believed to play a vital role in causing inflammation of the joints. Researchers believe they have identified an antibody which will block this disease-causing molecule. The drug is not a cure and it cannot reverse damage. Whether it remains effective over prolonged periods is uncertain, long-term side-effects are also unknown. However, a similar anti-TNF drug has had fantastic results in America. Pain levels have significantly dropped and the number of swollen and tender joints has been reduced. The drug has also dramatically helped to boost energy levels and banish tiredness.

There are fifteen places on the trial and the professor

running the trial wants candidates who have not responded to conventional medicine. Dr Campbell will be presenting my case in front of the professor and an audience of doctors and nurses. I watch fresh-faced doctors, nurses and medical students take their seats. The professor, dressed in a white coat, strides authoritatively into the room. Voices become muffled.

Dr Campbell begins. 'Ladies, gentlemen, this is Alice Peterson. She is twenty-four and has suffered from rheumatoid arthritis for six years and her case is very severe. She first came to see Dr Buckley in 1992 with symptoms of synovitis, tender hands and shoulders and her left knee was inflamed. Dr Buckley injected the knee with steroid and set her up on naproxen. At this stage Alice was planning to go to America, having been awarded a tennis scholarship.'

I am pleased he said that. It makes me feel more of a person.

'She has not yet, to date, responded to conventional treatment. We have put her on every drug under the sun – gold, methotrexate, cyclosporin, azathioprine, penicillamine, prednisolone, but she has had six years of constant pain, needles, injections, swelling, Baker's cysts, anaemia, raised hopes, thwarted hopes and major surgery. She has had operations on her hands and feet, a total hip replacement and is waiting for an ankle operation. She has had to watch her body change in the most appalling way.'

I look at the faces. One of the students smiles at me warmly, another smiles sympathetically, but Professor Madox looks like stone, expressionless – I can see no emotion in his face. Instead, he looks straight through me.

'Alice finished her degree at Bristol University two years ago and moved to London,' Dr Campbell continues, 'working part-time in a picture research library. However, the severity of her arthritis made it impossible for her to continue being independent. She is now back at home under the care of her parents. To be honest, I am stuck,' he says, looking pained himself. 'I think the only way forward is to try something new. We need fresh hope. Alice's RA is running away with itself, it will continue to cause more damage and more pain . . . that's a certainty. I think she has to take a risk and go on this trial. I know places are limited, but I cannot think of anyone else who should have higher priority.'

Dr Campbell finishes presenting my case.

Professor Madox begins to fire questions at me like a tennis-ball machine. 'Shut your eyes, tell me what is hurting most,' he says.

I wiggle my hands and feet.

'Don't move anything about,' he says sharply. 'Keep still, tell me what is hurting.'

'My ankle.'

'Where?'

'Around the subtalor joint, the heel. The ankle is agony when I walk.'

'But apart from that, nothing hurts?' he asks before I have the chance to tell him I have pain in the back of my head, my neck, my back, my knees, my feet, my hands . . .

'Do you feel tired?' he asks brusquely.

'Yes, most of the time.'

'Tiredness is a big issue then. Would you say you felt more tiredness without pain, or pain without tiredness?'

'I feel both. The tiredness comes with the pain.'

'Describe that pain.'

'I can't describe my pain,' I say, breathing deeply. 'All I can say is when I wake up I dread putting one foot in front of the other.'

'Can we see you walk?'

My hunched figure stands up gingerly. It takes me two to three minutes before I can start walking. It feels like I have broken glass in my foot. I begin to walk across the hall. My right ankle, I call it my wonky ankle, is so rolled over that it forces me to walk on the inside of my leg. It crunches like floorboards. I keep my head down, I don't want to see their reactions.

There is a moment of silence. It is a moment of understanding from the audience.

The professor's face suddenly appears more human. His voice softens. 'I am sorry to make you do that but I have to see if you qualify for the trial I'm running.'

'And do I?' I stammer desperately.

'Let's talk outside,' he says, getting up and marching out of the hall.

I follow slowly on the arm of Dr Campbell. 'It went well,' he smiles reassuringly.

We all sit down.

'You have a place, Alice,' the professor says without hesitation. 'The trial starts in four to eight weeks. If all goes to plan I'll look forward to seeing you then.'

Sixteen weeks later. The trial has begun. But I'm not on it. The licensing authority of the government said I could not enter the trial because I am of child-bearing age – they are concerned about the effects the drug could have on an unborn baby should I become pregnant now, or in the future. I am livid. How can they bring this into the equation? Anyway, how can I bring another life into the picture when I have no life? The priority is for me to get better before I can even think about little babies and, ultimately, it should be my choice to take the risk. I am an adult who can make adult decisions. My father, doggedly determined to get me on to the trial, wrote a strong letter on my behalf to the Secretary of State, Frank Dobson, arguing my case. We are pushing, harassing and waiting for a response although it feels like we are hitting our heads against a brick wall. We are all desperate.

It's now September. We have finally won the battle and I can begin the trial, seven long months after the initial start date. I simply need to undergo some tests beforehand – chest X-rays and blood tests.

'We'll get the results in two days, Alice,' says the sister, who is part of the Bath team working on the trial.

'What exactly are we testing for?'

'We have to check that your kidneys, liver and basically everything other than the RA is healthy before giving you the drug. It's routine. and I can't imagine that there will be a problem. I think you can firmly pencil in the first injection next week,' she says optimistically.

'At long last,' I say, breathing deeply. I like her, she's kind and understands how important this is to me.

Mum helps me to the car and we drive home, singing along to Mum's favourite car tape.

'Alice, hi,' the sister says ominously.

I sense immediately that something is wrong. 'Is there a problem?' I ask nervously.

'I hate to tell you this. I know how keen you are to start after all this time. Your blood test . . .'

'Yes,' I cut in. 'What's wrong?'

'Your liver function is surprisingly high and, until it comes down to the required level, you can't take part.'

'My liver function?' I ask, shocked. 'But I've never had problems before. Why now?'

'We don't know. None of us could believe it.'

I am sinking lower and lower and I can hardly breathe. I am biting my lip, trying not to cry.

'Alice, don't panic, love, we'll prescribe you another anti-inflammatory. The one you're on might be causing this problem. You'll need more blood tests until the level has gone down. It has to be below 84.'

'I'll have one tomorrow,' I suggest desperately.

'No, in a week's time, after taking the new anti-inflammatory.'

'But what happens if it doesn't go down?'

'It needs to be down by the end of the month because we can't recruit any more patients after the thirtieth.'

My desperation erupts like a volcano. I scream so loudly the walls almost shake. 'No,' I sob. 'No, no, no. Mum,' I pull weakly at her jumper. 'I should be on this drug. We fought for months to get me on the trial, I can't wait any longer,' I cry. 'I can't wait,' I scream. 'Mum, if I carry on like this I will die,' I say, crushing my head against the table. 'Please, God, give me a break. I will die,' I repeat, sobbing, screaming. Mum cannot find the right words to say and she leaves the room in tears. Dad's efforts to comfort me don't work this time either. I tell him fiercely that I want to be on my own. I tell him it's no use praying, or believing I will get better, and for a split, agonizing second I think he believes me.

★

'Granny,' I say, 'I'm sorry about my outburst.' Granny is staying with us and was so upset by the news that she went upstairs immediately and started to pack. I watch her move around the room, feeling for her belongings. She is now ninety-five and totally blind.

'My poor girl,' she says. 'I feel so bad for you and I'm an extra burden. I must go.'

'No, I'm sorry, I needed to shout and scream but I feel better now. We don't want you to go, Granny.'

'My dear Alice,' she says, finding my face and kissing me. 'I want to see you get better more than anything in the world.' Her blue eyes, which have seen so much in a lifetime, are crying. Granny may have lost her sight but she can see more clearly than ever.

'I'll have another blood test next week, Granny. It will be fine.'

'You brave, brave girl,' she says, looking into my face as if she can see me.

'Maybe I take after you,' I cry, hugging her tightly. 'I love you. Don't go.'

'Alice, it's gone down, but not enough,' the sister says a week later.

Another week of killing time crawls by. I am not sleeping, I am sick with worry. This is all I have to live for. Rebecca, Helen, friends and family ring and e-mail constantly, wanting to hear the latest update. I wish I was in touch with Sophie. We have not spoken since finals and I miss her friendship enormously.

'Hels, I'm scared I'm going to live like this all my life, that nothing will help. That this is it.'

'I'm scared for you too, but I can't help believing it will be OK, you've got to carry on hoping that you will

248

get on the trial,' Helen says on the other end of the line. I can picture her curled on the corner of her dark red sofa, in her rainbow-coloured flat, fresh flowers on the mantelpiece, a few candles lighting the night ahead. I long to press a button and be with her. She only has to hold my hand gently to cast me under her magical spell, where I feel safe and reassured under her umbrella of strength and hope. But I feel miles away from her.

'Alice, come on, you can't give up now. Don't you dare.' There is silence. I can hear her deeply inhaling her cigarette. My eyes are watering, my insides feel clogged with fear, an agonizing dread of the future.

'Al,' Helen says forcefully, 'just remember, the show ain't over till the fat lady sings. You've got to keep fighting this, right to the end.'

It's coming to the end of the month. This is my last chance, I think as my arm is pricked for more blood.

An agonizing twenty-four hours later, the sister rings. 'Alice, hi, how are you?'

Forget how I am. 'The results?'

'You got in by one point. You are now officially on the trial for a year,' she announces, almost as happy as I am.

'Oh, thank God,' I say, feeling every pore of my body open up and overflow with happiness and relief. 'When can I start?' I am shaking my head vigorously at Dad, who is hovering anxiously in the kitchen.

'Next week.'

As I put the phone down, Dad comes in and hugs me. I am laughing and crying with relief. No words will come out.

'We'll get there in the end,' Dad says. 'We'll get there.'

39

Placebo

The trial has begun. It involves one injection each week and check-ups each fortnight along with questionnaires, joint counts and blood tests. Today is my first injection day and I have to learn to inject myself. There are four drug strengths – 20mg, 40mg, 80mg, or placebo. Nobody knows which strength they are receiving. I am now terrified I will receive placebo, which means I will be injecting myself with a medication without active drug substance.

One in four patients receives placebo for the first twelve weeks and then receives the middle dose for the remaining year. I am a number on the trial and nobody can tell me whether I am the unfortunate placebo case, trundling down to Bath to have what I call the 'fucking unlucky' injection.

One of the trial doctors opens the card box with the two vials.

'It looks suspiciously like water,' I say to him. 'Oh no, I can't bear it. It's water. Placebo. I'm placebo. Do all the injections look like this, or is it just mine that looks like water?' I ask him. Perhaps I could have a little taste when his back is turned, but can you imagine how devastated I'd feel if it was water, especially after waiting months to get the drug?

'Oh, dear God, please not placebo,' Mum says.

'You are paranoid, the pair of you,' he says, smiling at us.

'No, only desperate. OK, what do I have to do?' I ask, rolling up my sleeves.

'Right, remove the metal cover from the top of the vial and give it a good clean with the alcohol wipe.'

I pick up the vial. The top's too stiff and I spend several minutes grappling with the little cap. Mum's laughing already. 'I can't do it, great start.'

'They are stiff,' he says. 'Give it to Nurse Mum, see if she can do it.'

'Oh lord, they are tight, oh goodness . . .' Finally, she succeeds and the first step is over.

'Now the hard bit, inserting needle into vial. I find that wiggling the cap is the best way to get the cover off the needle. Like this.' He shows me. 'Now you try.'

'It's too stiff, my hands are hopeless.'

'Wiggle it, wiggle it . . .' he's saying.

'I am wiggling.' There's a crunching sound. 'Don't worry, that was only my shoulder,' I say, now laughing uncontrollably with nerves.

The sister pops her head round the door. 'It sounds as if you are having a party in here, I've never heard anything like it!'

The cover is finally off and the needle wobbles towards the vial. I stick it in with trembling hands as Mum laughs at me. 'Mum, please go away, you're not making this any easier!'

We are finally ready to inject and I have the lovely choice of either the thigh or the abdomen. I opt for the thigh.

'Point the needle down and plunge it in, almost like a dart,' he says.

The needle is wavering like a drunkard towards my thigh.

It's in. It stings. I shut my eyes. 'Dear God, please not placebo,' I pray for the millionth time.

40

Today . . .

Things that I love:

- A Clarins facial.
- Hydrotherapy.
- All the helpers and physios at the hydrotherapy centre.
- Watching *Friends* – have developed a huge crush on Chandler.
- Writing – I'm working on book number two . . .
- My Duxiana double bed with goose-down duvet.
- Good-looking doctors, I must marry one.
- Pulling silly faces at Mum.
- Watching Dad try to set the video recorder.
- Eating 'Go Ahead!' 85 per cent fat-free strawberry creams and Sainsbury's Indulgence Toffee Nut explosion ice-cream.
- e-mail – can now be in touch with friends constantly.
- My rusty wheelchair collecting dust.
- Researchers and scientists who are working towards a cure for arthritis.
- Vodka and tonic.
- Flying kites.
- Watching Tim Henman.
- Ticking, 'without ANY difficulty'!
- Screening calls.
- Meeting other people with RA or similar conditions, and sharing experiences.

- Helen painting my toes silver.
- Cousin Emma's chicken with lemon and ten cloves of garlic.
- Playing cards with Emma's gorgeous children, Jamie and Archie.
- Seeing my grandmother, blind and now aged ninety-seven, who is one of the most courageous, inspiring people I know.
- Friends (not the television programme this time!).
- Seeing Sophie again and rebuilding our friendship.
- Hot-water bottles.
- Furry zebra-striped slippers.
- Surgeons who perform miraculous operations.
- Occupational therapists and physiotherapists.
- Hearing Tom's infectious laugh.
- Shopping at Whistles.
- Drawstring trousers.
- My independence.
- The Bath trial team.
- MY MAGIC DRUG.

Three months into the trial and my life has changed dramatically. A reflection I hardly recognize smiles back at me in the mirror, a reflection that is full of life. I am still in pain, but the pain is tolerable, and I know that I will have to tackle problems ahead. But my weekly injection is letting me live. Life is no longer a dark, black tunnel, where everything I do is tinged with its blackness. A new life with different challenges is waiting to be explored. Like an imprisoned bird with damaged wings, I have been set free to fly. I move forward, leaving my past behind, and the sad memories are beginning to fade.

Everyone deals with illness and pain in different ways,

there is no set pattern. However, I have learnt that hiding behind my illness, and not seeing how it affects other people, can cause terrible heartache. With Sophie and the flatmates, I was not ready to accept that I was not quite the same as them, that I needed extra help and care that they could not provide during finals. If I could rewind time, I would do things differently and I am so sorry to have lost important friendships which, after three years, I have the chance to rebuild. Although, maybe, I had to go through that stage to get to where I am now.

My book has brought back all the happy memories of my tennis. I relived those moments in my heart and my love for tennis has finally been revived.

I am glad I never gave up. I am happy. Deep down I have not changed. I am still Alice. I am still young. And I'm still here.

Hope is a life-giving force. For those struggling in the dark, don't ever lose sight of it. It's what will bring you back into the world of light.

'Right, I'm ready,' I call, looking at all my bags and suitcases piled up in the boot and back seat of the car.

Mum holds me closely. 'I'll miss you so much,' she says. 'The house will be quiet without you.'

'It will be lovely,' I smile. 'Just you and Dad, and you can begin to play golf again!'

Mum is not afraid of showing her tears. 'You've lost that awful look of pain which masked your lovely face,' she tells me, holding my cheeks in her warm hands.

'Mum,' I say, knowing I'm about to cry. I hate emotional goodbyes.

'I mean it,' she perseveres. 'Your eyes are alive, it's like you've been born again.' She kisses me. 'You're my precious girl.'

Dad stands quietly, absorbing everything we are saying. When Mum eventually lets go he takes over.

'Sod it,' I say, hugging him. 'I'll miss you, old man.'

He hugs me tightly. 'Cheeky girl. I love you,' he says.

I knew how hard this day would be, despite both myself and my parents wishing for this moment for so long.

'I've got to go now, you know how I hate goodbyes,' I say, sitting down behind the wheel, starting the engine. A tape is slotted in and I wind down the window to give Mum and Dad one more kiss. 'Thank you for everything,' I say to them, my tearful voice trying not to break. I drive off quickly, watching the figures of my parents in the back mirror.

There they stand, next to each other like one unique tree of strength and love. How fortunate I am to be able to lean on it, its roots staying firm, its branches protecting and supporting me.

London! A new life! Back with friends! A new beginning! A new me! I feel excited by the future. I want to make up for lost time and travel. I want to go to Africa to see Granny's old home and see the giraffes and the elephants. I want to meet someone and fall head over heels in love. I want to carry on writing. I suddenly grin widely, realizing I have just cracked the new title for my book. And on that happy thought my car turns another corner . . .

Epilogue

Since writing, *A Will to Win* I have moved to west London. I rent a mews flat. It's in a wonderful location, near to the Portobello market. In between writing breaks I find myself in lethal shops like Jigsaw and I can feed myself cheaply on the fruit and vegetables from the market. I live on my own, so being in a mews is ideal because I am surrounded by people. I have a great French neighbour who doesn't mind opening bottles for me or scrambling on chairs to put light bulbs in. It was a big daunting step finally to move away from home. I miss Mum, Dad, and even Jasmine, my miniature dachshund. I miss the goings-on at home and there are times when I wish I could press a button to be back. But I have made that important break now and I value my independence. I don't rely on my parents the way I used to. I get myself to places on my own. I cook for myself and friends. I have my own answer machine. I do my own ironing and buy loo rolls – things that I've longed to do! When Mum comes to stay I am proud that she's staying in *my* home.

I have converted one of the rooms into an office with a large glass desk to scatter my files, books and paper. I am continuing to work on my second book which I plan to finish this year. This is a follow-on to *A Will to Win*, in that I am continuing to share with the reader how I am and my hopes and dreams for the future. A few of the family and friends from *A Will to Win* reappear in this book too. It describes how I set out to learn more about my grandmother's pioneering life in Africa. As the story unfolds I learn where so much of my strength, and my mother's, to fight the RA has come from. Granny is now ninety-eight, blind and an inspiration to me. As a young woman, she had the courage to leave her home – she was brought up in a castle – and family behind, and the determination to start a new life in Africa. In January 2000, I travelled to Zimbabwe with my mother and aunt to visit her old home. Helen and her boyfriend James came out for a week. Dad also joined us for the last two weeks, dressed in his woolly jumper and scarf.

The travelling was a challenge, but one I would have never even contemplated before the drug trial. My doctor was happy to let me administer my magic drug while away, as long as I remembered to put it in the fridge wherever I was. I found the travelling tough and at that stage my recently operated-on ankle was at times so painful that I couldn't walk. Then there were moments of pride when I managed to climb, with my ankle splint firmly strapped on, up the Matopos to Rhodes's grave. Yet one of the best things about the trip was being at Granny's old home, feeling close to her story and being able to imagine the life she led. Towards the end of our holiday we went to a few safari lodges. The guides would gently lift me into the safari jeeps without even questioning why I couldn't get up on my own. It was a dream fulfilled to see so many giraffes, lions and elephants.

My magic drug still works. I am on a fortnightly injection and have check-ups every two months. However, there are still many obstacles ahead. I am currently on the waiting list to have a hip replaced. My friends call me the bionic woman. My magic drug takes a great deal of the pain away but unfortunately it's not a cure. Nothing can reverse the damage already done to my joints. That's what still causes the pain and restricts my mobility. I can't walk far without feeling tired or sore. It's invaluable having a car because I find buses and tubes impossible. Buses never give me enough time to get off and the tube is only OK if I don't need to make changes. If I was rich I'd get black cabs all the time, although at times even they are difficult to get in and out of! It is hard at times and there are always moments when I scream or cry with frustration. I have to be unafraid to ask for help. That's what makes life possible.

Being back in London has helped me to stay in touch with friends. Sophie and I have slowly rebuilt our friendship. After the raw break-up it took us three years before we made contact. We had to get to know one another again. Our relationship has changed in that I don't depend on her for support in the way I used to. We still confide in one another and support each other in our work and relationships. But all the fun and laughter we shared has come back again. We have an understanding that our friendship will never get pushed to the extreme of finals at Bristol. She is about to go to Madrid for a year to teach. I will miss her desperately, especially our evenings talking over a bowl of olives and a glass of wine. I am already planning my flight out. Thank God for email . . .

I have met many friends through Sophie and I continue to see my Bristol friends who are now in London. Matthew still runs marathons for ARC. Rebecca is in London and works for a design company. I spend a lot of time with Rebecca and her sister. I occasionally see Seb, which is lovely. I have also met a few new friends, a couple of whom I met through my work at the art library in west London. Writing is a solitary occupation and I do get lonely. To break up the day I go swimming. I like to think it keeps me slim and fit. I also like to do as much as I can in the evenings, either eating out or having people over to my flat – something I missed when I was at home. I enjoy doing all the normal things again like going to the cinema and going to parties. A friend and I also love Art 4 Fun, where we pick out something to paint which gets fired and glazed. I find it really therapeutic.

My sister, Helen, is about to buy a house in Shepherds Bush which is a relief for me as I will not have to stagger four flights of stairs to get to her front door. She married James Noel in January 2001. I was proud to be her bridesmaid and wore an Amanda Wakely dress! It was a long slim-fitting silver dress and I felt so sexy! When I put it on I could not believe something could make me feel so good. I hadn't felt like it for a long time. Helen is expecting a baby girl early next year. She continues to be a wonderful support. My linchpin. She works from home too, so we often spend time together during the day. I work upstairs with my laptop; she is downstairs on her computer. With her support I can stay in London for about two weeks before I am aching to be at home. I need a couple of days to rest before I feel ready to go back. When away from home, my parents are always on the end of the phone, the bills are enormous. Mum continues to make lampshades; Dad still says, 'Sod it.'

I have lived in London for eighteen months and I can't see myself being anywhere else right now. It's where my friends are. Also I think it's a stimulating place to live – there's always an art exhibition, a new play or concert to go to. Or a new restaurant to try out. And great shops. I try not to let myself worry about the future but live each day, one at a time. There are still times when the pain depresses me and I wonder what life is all about. I'm scared about my forthcoming hip operation and have needed to see Jenny again. Above all, my writing helps me. Life has been exciting since the launch of *A Will to Win*. My family and friends gathered together for a party to celebrate the beginning of something new. It has opened more doors. I am currently involved in touring the country, giving talks to audiences that range from the general public to those in the medical profession. I want to continue to raise the profile of RA, particularly in relation to how it affects the lives of the young.

Alice Peterson
October 2001